Women's Neurology

WHAT DO I DO NOW?

SERIES CO-EDITORS-IN-CHIEF
Lawrence C. Newman, MD
Director, Brain Health
Atria Institute
Professor of Neurology
New York University Langone Health
New York, New York

Morris Levin, MD
Director of the Headache Center
Professor of Neurology
University of California, San Francisco
San Francisco, California

OTHER VOLUMES IN THE SERIES

Epilepsy
Pain
Neuroinfections
Neurogenetics
Neurotology
Pediatric Neurology, Second Edition
Stroke, Second Edition
Peripheral Nerve and Muscle Disease, Second Edition
Cerebrovascular Disease, Second Edition
Movement Disorders, Second Edition
Neuroimmunology, Second Edition
Neuro-Ophthalmology, Second Edition
Concussion
Emergency Neurology, Second Edition
Headache and Facial Pain, Second Edition
Neurocritical Care, Third Edition

Women's Neurology

SECOND EDITION

Edited by

Lena G. Liu, MD
Mass General Brigham

and

Christina R. Catherine, MD, PhD
University of Pittsburgh Medical Center

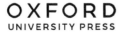

OXFORD
UNIVERSITY PRESS

Oxford University Press is a department of the University of Oxford.
It furthers the University's objective of excellence in research, scholarship,
and education by publishing worldwide. Oxford is a registered trade mark of
Oxford University Press in the UK and certain other countries.

Published in the United States of America by Oxford University Press
198 Madison Avenue, New York, NY 10016, United States of America.

© Oxford University Press 2025

All rights reserved. No part of this publication may be reproduced, stored in a retrieval system, transmitted, used for text and data mining, or used for training artificial intelligence, in any form or by any means, without the prior permission in writing of Oxford University Press, or as expressly permitted by law, by license or under terms agreed with the appropriate reprographics rights organization. Inquiries concerning reproduction outside the scope of the above should be sent to the Rights Department, Oxford University Press, at the address above.

You must not circulate this work in any other form
and you must impose this same condition on any acquirer

Library of Congress Cataloging-in-Publication Data
Names: Liu, Lena G., editor. | Catherine, Christina R. (Christina Rose), editor.
Title: Women's neurology / edited by Lena G. Liu and Christina R. Catherine.
Other titles: What do I do now?
Description: 2 edition. | New York, NY : Oxford University Press, [2025] |
Series: What do i do now | Includes bibliographical references and index.
Identifiers: LCCN 2024044157 | ISBN 9780197749722 (paperback) | ISBN 9780197749746 (epub) |
ISBN 9780197749739 (updf) | ISBN 9780197749753 (online)
Subjects: MESH: Nervous System Diseases—diagnosis | Nervous System Diseases—therapy |
Women | Case Reports Classification: LCC RC451.4.W6 | NLM WL 140 |
DDC 616.80082—dc23/eng/20241118
LC record available at https://lccn.loc.gov/2024044157

This material is not intended to be, and should not be considered, a substitute for medical or other professional advice. Treatment for the conditions described in this material is highly dependent on the individual circumstances. And, while this material is designed to offer accurate information with respect to the subject matter covered and to be current as of the time it was written, research and knowledge about medical and health issues is constantly evolving and dose schedules for medications are being revised continually, with new side effects recognized and accounted for regularly. Readers must therefore always check the product information and clinical procedures with the most up-to-date published product information and data sheets provided by the manufacturers and the most recent codes of conduct and safety regulation. The publisher and the authors make no representations or warranties to readers, express or implied, as to the accuracy or completeness of this material. Without limiting the foregoing, the publisher and the authors make no representations or warranties as to the accuracy or efficacy of the drug dosages mentioned in the material. The authors and the publisher do not accept, and expressly disclaim, any responsibility for any liability, loss or risk that may be claimed or incurred as a consequence of the use and/ or application of any of the contents of this material.

DOI: 10.1093/med/9780197749722.001.0001

Printed by Marquis Book Printing, Canada

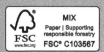

Contents

Contributors ix

SECTION I: SEIZURES AND EPILEPSY 1

1. **Seizures Occurring Once a Month** 3
   Lena G. Liu

2. **Pain in the Back** 7
   M. Angela O'Neal and Emily L. Johnson

3. **A Young Woman With Jerking Movements** 11
   Christina R. Catherine and Wesley T. Kerr

4. **Functional Neurologic Symptoms** 23
   Emily L. Johnson

5A. **A Young Woman With Epilepsy and PCOS** 29
   M. Angela O'Neal, Revised by Caroline Just, Ginette Moores,
   and Esther Bui

5B. **A Young Woman With Epilepsy and Family Planning** 33
   M. Angela O'Neal, Revised by Caroline Just, Ginette Moores,
   and Esther Bui

6. **Frequent Seizures During Pregnancy** 39
   Christina R. Catherine and Alexandra Urban

SECTION II: AUTOIMMUNE AND PARANEOPLASTIC DISORDERS 45

7. **Multiple Sclerosis** 47
   Sarah Conway and Tamara B. Kaplan

8. **A Mother Who Could Not See Her Baby** 59
   Sarah Conway and Tamara B. Kaplan

9. **Myelin Oligodendrocyte Glycoprotein Antibody-Associated Disease** 65
   Sarah Conway and Tamara B. Kaplan

10. **Autoimmune Encephalitis** 71
    Sarah Conway and Tamara B. Kaplan

11. **Paraneoplastic Cerebellar Degeneration** 75
Sarah Conway and Tamara B. Kaplan

SECTION III: HEADACHE DISORDERS 79

12. **Hormonal Contraception in a Woman With Headache** 81
Addie Peretz

13. **Headache Around Menses** 89
Addie Peretz, Regina Krel, and Paul G. Mathew

14. **Seeing Spots: Complicated Migraines** 95
Christina R. Catherine

15. **Headaches: When It's Not a Migraine** 101
Arathi Nandyala and Addie Peretz

16. **A Woman With a Headache in the Second Trimester** 111
Christina R. Catherine

17. **Acute Headache in Pregnancy** 119
M. Angela O'Neal and Addie Peretz

18. **Chiari Malformation in Pregnancy** 125
Janet F. R. Waters

19. **The Worst Headache of Her Life** 129
Alison Seitz and Eliza Miller

20. **Postpartum Left-Sided Numbness and Right-Sided Shaking** 133
Alison Seitz and Eliza Miller

SECTION IV: STROKE AND VASCULAR DISORDERS 137

21. **A Pregnant Woman With Aphasia and Right-Sided Weakness** 139
Alison Seitz and Eliza Miller

22. **"Will I Have a Stroke?"** 145
Alison Seitz and Eliza Miller

SECTION V: NEUROMUSCULAR DISORDERS AND NEUROPATHIES 149

23. **A Young Woman With Double Vision and Fatigue** 151
Carolina Barnett-Tapia and Vera Bril

24. **Pregnancy in Women With Hereditary/Genetic Myopathies** 159
Dubravka Dodig and Mark Tarnopolsky

25. **Numbness in the Hand of a Woman During Pregnancy** 169
Carolina Barnett-Tapia

26. **A Woman With Leg Weakness After Delivery** 175
Nouf Alfaidi and Carolina Barnett-Tapia

SECTION VI: NEURO-INFECTIOUS DISEASE 183

27. **"I Can't Concentrate at Work"** 185
Caleb R. S. McEntire, George K. Harrold, and Kathleen Miller

28. **A Woman With Headache and Confusion** 195
Caleb R. S. McEntire and Miriam B. Barshak

29. **"I Can't Concentrate Anymore"** 205
Caleb R. S. McEntire and Howard M. Heller

30. **COVID-19 Neurologic Complications During Pregnancy** 213
Christina R. Catherine

SECTION VII: NEURO-ONCOLOGY 219

31. **Newlywed With Headache, Morning Sickness, and Right-Sided Weakness** 221
Varun Jain and Kevin B. Elmore

SECTION VIII: NEURO-OPHTHALMOLOGY 227

32. **A Woman With Painful Blurry Vision** 229
Islam Zaydan

33. **Painless Loss of Vision** 235
Islam Zaydan

34. **New-Onset Headache With Vision Changes in an Elderly Woman** 241
Islam Zaydan

SECTION IX: MOVEMENT DISORDERS 247

35. **Parkinson's Disease in Women** 249
Veronica Bruno and Elizabeth Slow

36. **Huntington Disease** 259
Jane Liao and Elizabeth Slow

37. **An Irresistible Urge to Move** 265
Sanskriti Sasikumar

38. **The Elderly Woman With Shaky Hands** 273
Elizabeth Slow

39. **Chorea Gravidarum** 279
Laura Armengou-Garcia and Elizabeth Slow

SECTION X: COGNITIVE AND BEHAVIORAL NEUROLOGY 285

40. **A Woman With Cognitive Concerns** 287
M. Angela O'Neal and Sara C. LaHue

41. **Memory Concerns in Middle Age** 291
Sara C. LaHue and Marie Pasinski

SECTION XI: PREGNANCY-RELATED AND PERIPARTUM-RELATED CONDITIONS 299

42. **Neurological Complications of Hypertensive Disorders of Pregnancy** 301
Kristine Brown, Whitney Booker, and Eliza Miller

43. **Third-Trimester Headache, Hypertension, and Seizure** 307
Kristine Brown, Whitney Booker, and Eliza Miller

44. **A Woman With Severe Headache and Visual Disturbances Postpartum** 311
Kristine Brown, Whitney Booker, and Eliza Miller

45. **A Woman in Labor With Hypotension and Dyspnea After Epidural Placement** 315
Janet F. R. Waters and Jonathan H. Waters

46. **Ringing in the Ears and Pain in the Head** 321
M. Angela O'Neal, Janet F. R. Waters, and Jonathan H. Waters

    Index 327

Contributors

Nouf Alfaidi, MBBS
University of Toronto

Laura Armengou-Garcia, MD
University of Toronto

**Carolina Barnett-Tapia,
MD, PhD**
University of Toronto

Miriam B. Barshak, MD
Harvard Medical School,
Massachusetts General Hospital

Whitney Booker, MD
Columbia University
Medical Center

Vera Bril, MD
University of Toronto

Kristine Brown, MD
Columbia University
Medical Center

Veronica Bruno, MD, MPH
University of Calgary

Esther Bui, MD, FRCPC
University of Toronto

**Christina R. Catherine,
MD, PhD**
University of Pittsburgh
Medical Center

Sarah Conway, MD
Brigham and Women's Hospital,
Harvard Medical School

Dubravka Dodig, MD
University of Toronto

Kevin B. Elmore, MD
Mount Sinai Hospital

George K. Harrold, MD
Harvard Medical School

Howard M. Heller, MD, MPH
Harvard Medical School

Varun Jain, MBBS
Mount Sinai Hospital

Emily L. Johnson, MD, MPH
Johns Hopkins School of Medicine

Caroline Just, MD, FRCPC
Cleveland Clinic Lerner College
of Medicine,
Case Western Reserve University

Tamara B. Kaplan, MD
Brigham and Women's Hospital

Wesley T. Kerr, MD, PhD
University of Pittsburgh

Regina Krel, MD, FAHS
Hackensack University
Medical Center

Sara C. LaHue, MD
University of California, San Francisco

Jane Liao, MD, MSc
University of Toronto

Lena G. Liu, MD
Mass General Brigham

Paul G. Mathew, MD, DNBPAS, FAAN, FAHS
Harvard Medical School

Caleb R. S. McEntire, MD
Harvard Medical School

Eliza Miller, MD, MS
Columbia University Medical Center

Kathleen Miller, MD
Harvard Medical School

Ginette Moores, MD, FRCPC, CSCN
University of Toronto

Arathi Nandyala, MD
Stanford Health Care

M. Angela O'Neal, MD
Mass General Brigham

Marie Pasinski, MD
Mass General Brigham

Addie Peretz, MD
Stanford University

Sanskriti Sasikumar, MD
University of Toronto

Alison Seitz, MD
University of Washington

Elizabeth Slow, MD, PhD
University of Toronto

Mark Tarnopolsky, MD, PhD
McMaster University

Alexandra Urban, MD
University of Pittsburgh Medical Center

Janet F. R. Waters, MD, MBA
University of Pittsburgh Medical Center

Jonathan H. Waters, MD
University of Pittsburgh Medical Center

Islam Zaydan, MD
University of Pittsburgh Medical Center

SECTION I

Seizures and Epilepsy

1 Seizures Occurring Once a Month

Lena G. Liu

A 36-year-old woman is referred for evaluation for epilepsy, which had started one year previously. Her boyfriend, who had witnessed many of the seizures, described them as beginning with lip smacking, followed by repetitive movements of her left hand. The patient would stare blankly ahead and not respond appropriately to questioning. This was followed in half the cases by a tonic posture with arms flexed and legs extended and then brief clonic movements. The seizures were usually 1–2 minutes in duration and followed by a postictal confusion lasting up to 15 minutes. She usually has three or four focal impaired awareness seizures per month, typically at the onset of her menses. These secondarily generalize approximately once per month, also around the onset of her menses. Her menses are regular. She is currently on levetiracetam 750 mg twice daily. Brain MRI was normal. Her electroencephalogram was also normal. Her exam is normal.

What do you do now?

CATAMENIAL EPILEPSY

Hormones can alter seizure frequency through modulation of brain excitability as well as through their effect on anticonvulsant drug concentrations. Animal studies have suggested that estrogen is a proconvulsant through the mechanism of decreased chloride ion conductance at $GABA_A$ receptors, whereas progesterone, particularly its metabolite allopregnanolone, promotes neuroinhibition and acts as an anticonvulsant through the mechanism of increased chloride ion conductance at $GABA_A$ receptors.[1]

Catamenial epilepsy is defined as the cyclic exacerbation of seizures in relation to the menstrual cycle. A catamenial pattern may be seen with any type of epilepsy, but it is more common with focal epilepsies. Using the definition that there is a doubling of seizure frequency associated with a particular phase of the menstrual cycle, up to one-third of women have catamenial epilepsy. A diagnosis of catamenial epilepsy is made after careful assessment of menstrual and seizure diaries across at least three menstrual cycles.

A normal menstrual cycle is 28 days, with day 1 defined as the first day of menses, and day 14 defined as the day of ovulation. The first half of the menstrual cycle, days 1–14, is called the *follicular phase*; the second half, days −14 to −1, is called the *luteal phase*. Different patterns of catamenial epilepsy have been described. The most common type, as demonstrated by this patient, is the perimenstrual exacerbation (C1). This corresponds to a progesterone decline, which mimics a withdrawal of benzodiazepines and decreases the seizure threshold. The next most common pattern is the periovulatory exacerbation (C2). This is characterized by an increase in seizure frequency associated with ovulation and the associated surge in estrogen. The inadequate luteal pattern (C3) is the least frequent pattern. In this pattern, seizure frequency increases in the luteal phase of the menstrual cycle. This is associated with relatively low progesterone levels and anovulatory cycles due to abnormal follicle-stimulating hormone (FSH) secretion and subsequent poor development of a mature follicle and corpus luteum.[2] Thus, the maldeveloped corpus luteum secretes less progesterone than it should, whereas estrogen levels are not affected. The increased estrogen-to-progesterone ratio increases the seizure frequency during the luteal phase for women with a C3 pattern of catamenial epilepsy.

Most treatments have focused on the C1 pattern. Acetazolamide at doses of 250–500 mg daily, 3–7 days before menses, has been shown to be efficacious. Benzodiazepines have also been used especially for seizure clusters. The only benzodiazepine proven to have efficacy is clobazam. In a randomized controlled trial, clobazam was shown to be more effective than placebo. A trial with cyclic progesterone lozenges was ineffective in women with intractable focal seizures. However, there was a benefit for the subgroup of women with the C1 pattern who had greater than three times exacerbation of their seizures during the perimenstrual days.[3] The final strategy useful for C1 and C2 patterns would be to increase the antiseizure medication (ASM) dose during the phase of the catamenial exacerbation.[4] For women with a C3 pattern, which is often anovulatory and linked with irregular menses, cyclic and intermittent interventions are not an option. Therefore, the goal of treatment for those with a C3 pattern is long-term menstrual suppression with either combination oral contraceptive pills (OCPs) or medroxyprogesterone acetate, which provide a stable hormonal milieu and reduce unpredictable cyclic hormonal variation.[5]

KEY POINTS TO REMEMBER

- Many women have a catamenial exacerbation of their epilepsy, with up to one-third of women with epilepsy being affected.
- Defining the specific catamenial pattern is an important step in deciding on treatment strategy.
- Acetazolamide, clobazam, and cyclic progesterone lozenges, for the C1 pattern only, are effective in suppressing the catamenial seizure exacerbation. An alternative approach would be to increase the antiseizure medication (ASM) dose during the time of exacerbation.
- For the C3 pattern, the goal is long-term menstrual suppression with either combination oral contraceptive pills (OCPs) or medroxyprogesterone acetate, which provide a stable hormonal milieu and reduce unpredictable cyclic hormonal variation.

References

1. Harden CL, Pennell PB. Neuroendocrine considerations in the treatment of men and women with epilepsy. *Lancet Neurol.* 2013;12(1):72–83.

2. Herzog AG, Klein P, Ransil BJ. Three patterns of catamenial epilepsy. *Epilepsia.* 1997;38:1082–1088.

3. Herzog AG. Catamenial epilepsy: Update on prevalence, pathophysiology and treatment from the findings of the NIH Progesterone Treatment Trial. *Seizure.* 2015;28:18–25.

4. Pennell PB. Pregnancy, epilepsy, and women's issues. *Continuum.* 2013;19(3):697–714.

5. Navis A, Harden C. A treatment approach to catamenial epilepsy. *Curr Treat Options Neurol.* 2016;18(7):30.

2 Pain in the Back

M. Angela O'Neal and Emily L. Johnson

A 56-year-old woman is referred for evaluation of focal with secondary generalized epilepsy. She has a long history of epilepsy since her teens. Her seizures typically consist of staring with some lip smacking, following which she is confused and sleepy for 10 minutes. Occasionally, the seizures progress to bilateral tonic–clonic movements and a more prolonged confusional period of 20–30 minutes. She has been on a stable dose of carbamazepine for many years. Her brain MRI is normal, and a past electroencephalogram showed occasional right temporal sharp waves. Her last seizure was more than 1 year ago, in the setting of missing several doses of carbamazepine.

While carrying a heavy box, she developed severe low back pain. Her internist did a lumbar spine film, which showed an L1 compression fracture.

Her only medication is carbamazepine extended-release 400 mg twice per day.

Her back exam shows point tenderness at L1. Her neurologic exam is normal.

What do you do now?

EFFECTS OF NEUROLOGICAL DRUGS ON BONE HEALTH

Osteoporosis is a skeletal disorder in which decreased bone strength leads to fractures. Antiseizure medications (ASMs) are known to affect bone metabolism. This is especially true for those that induce the cytochrome P450 system. Activation of the P450 system causes increased breakdown of vitamin D. This in turn leads to less gastrointestinal absorption of calcium, which stimulates elevated levels of parathyroid hormone. Parathyroid hormone increases lead to more calcium mobilization from bone and increased bone turnover.[1]

Specific ASMs and Bone Health
The enzyme-inducing ASMs (EI-ASMs) include phenytoin, carbamazepine, phenobarbital, primidone, oxcarbazepine, eslicarbazepine, and cenobamate. Valproate is not an enzyme inducer. However, it is reported to increase both the rate of bone loss and fracture incidence. This appears to be correlated with dose and duration of valproate therapy. Clonazepam also has an associated small increased risk of fractures, whereas long-term topiramate use is associated with increased bone turnover. Studies on lamotrigine, levetiracetam, and zonisamide have demonstrated no adverse effects on bone mineral density.[2–4]

Risk Factors for Osteoporosis
Risk factors for osteoporosis have been well studied. They include female sex, postmenopausal state, inactivity, low body mass, chronic illness, inadequate vitamin D and calcium intake, limited sunlight exposure, and smoking. Additional risk factors for osteoporosis in patients with epilepsy include the type and number of ASMs and the duration of therapy.

Epilepsy and Fall Risk
Patients with epilepsy have a higher fall risk, both directly due to the epilepsy and due to the ASM effect on gait stability. This is especially true for individuals who have generalized epilepsy and those on multiple-drug regimens. In the Woman's Health Initiative study, which followed women ages 50–79 years on ASMs and those not on an ASM, the use of ASMs was clearly associated with a significant increase in risk of fractures. Fracture risk

is related to the epilepsy type; the degree of control of the epilepsy; and the drug regimen, including which ASMs are used, their dose, and the duration of therapy.[4]

Screening

Osteoporosis screening with a bone mineral density scan (BMD) is recommended for postmenopausal women and those with additional risk factors. In women with epilepsy, the risks of ASM use as well as the risks related to falls put them at even higher risk. It is reasonable to screen with a BMD in women with epilepsy who have additional risk factors for osteoporosis. In people with epilepsy on an ASM, it is recommended to periodically monitor serum calcium, phosphate, and 25-hydroxy vitamin D levels.[5]

Prevention

The usual lifestyle recommendations should also be made: regular weight-bearing exercise and smoking cessation. Low calcium or vitamin D levels should be replaced. Adequate calcium doses in older adults, 1,200 mg daily, and vitamin D 400–800 U daily, are recommended. Decisions surrounding changing an ASM regimen need to be individualized and weighed against the risk of recurrent seizure; when possible, changing an EI-ASM to a non-EI-ASM should be considered in women with long-term EI-ASM use with low bone density. Osteoporosis identified through BMD or after fractures may warrant treatment with a bisphosphonate to improve bone density.[6]

KEY POINTS TO REMEMBER

- ASMs, particularly those that are enzyme-inducing, increase the risk of osteoporosis.
- Patients with epilepsy have a higher fall risk.
- Patients at risk for osteoporosis should be screened with a BMD.
- Both calcium and vitamin D supplementation are important in patients with epilepsy to support bone health.

References

1. Pack AM. Bone disease in epilepsy. *Curr Neurol Neurosci Rep.* 2004;4:329–334.
2. Pack AM, Morrell MJ, Marcus R, et al. Bone mass and turnover in women with epilepsy on antiepileptic drug monotherapy. *Ann Neurol.* 2005;57:252–257.
3. Mintzer S, Boppana P, Toguri J, DeSantis A. Vitamin D levels and bone turnover in epilepsy patients taking carbamazepine or oxcarbazepine. *Epilepsia.* 2006;47:510–515.
4. Koo DL, Nam H. Effects of zonisamide monotherapy on bone health in drug-naïve epilepsy patients. *Epilepsia.* 2020;61:2142–2149.
5. Vestergaard P, Tigaran S, Rejnmark L, et al. Fracture risk is increased in epilepsy. *Acta Neurol Scand.* 1999;99:269–275.
6. Meier C, Kraenzlin ME. Antiepileptics and bone health. *Ther Adv Musculoskelet Dis.* 2011;3(5):235–243.

3 A Young Woman With Jerking Movements

Christina R. Catherine and

Wesley T. Kerr

A 20-year-old woman presents for evaluation of seizures. She had episodic jerking movements during the past year. These jerks seem to be correlated with times when she gets poor sleep. She was recently seen in the emergency department (ED) after blacking out. She had stayed up late studying for a final. She woke up, experienced several of these jerks, and then "blacked out." Her roommate found her on the floor and called an ambulance. She denied any tongue bite or incontinence but notes being sore and "foggy" when she woke up. The ED physician ordered a brain MRI, which was normal, and an electroencephalogram (EEG) shows 3- or 4-Hz generalized spike/polyspike and wave discharges. Neurological exam is normal. She takes fluoxetine and combined oral contraception.

What do you do now?

This case raises some of the important points to consider when choosing an antiseizure medication (ASM) for potential mothers, and it reviews the most frequently encountered generalized-onset epilepsies (GEs).

GENERALIZED-ONSET EPILEPSIES

Generalized-onset epilepsies are believed to cause approximately 30% of epilepsy across the lifespan and up to 20% of all adult epilepsies.[1] They are characterized by the absence of a clear structural brain abnormality on standard MRI; normal or near normal neurological examination and cognitive screening; and seizures beginning at certain age ranges.[1] Among children with new-onset epilepsy, 23–43% have GE, of which 53–58% have one of the four common idiopathic GEs: childhood absence epilepsy (CAE), juvenile absence epilepsy (JAE), juvenile myoclonic epilepsy (JME), or epilepsy with generalized-onset tonic–clonic seizures alone (EGTCS).[2] These four GEs affect 0.1% of the entire adult population and most often have a polygenic mode of inheritance.[3] Although less common, generalized-onset epilepsy with eyelid myoclonia is also a well-described condition. These five epilepsy syndromes are discussed in more detail below, including clinical presentations.

Treatment recommendations for the GEs are similar across different disorders. First-line treatment options include valproic acid and lamotrigine; second-line options include topiramate, zonisamide, levetiracetam, and benzodiazepines such as clobazam. Valproic acid and topiramate are generally avoided in people planning a pregnancy given the potential for teratogenicity. Valproic acid also has a multitude of potential side effects, including polycystic ovarian syndrome and weight gain, which in turn can lead to infertility. For people with epilepsy planning pregnancy, the use of levetiracetam, lamotrigine, or both is the preferred option, with the understanding that lamotrigine may worsen myoclonic jerks.[4] Brivaracetam and lacosamide may be an alternative option, although data are currently limited on its safety during pregnancy. In select situations, low-dose valproic acid (<625 mg total daily dose) may be used given patient preference after discussion of the potential teratogenic risks versus concern for seizure exacerbation.[5] In people with epilepsy who have a low or no likelihood of pregnancy (hysterectomy, tubal ligation, no sexual contact with sperm-producing people), valproic acid is an appropriate treatment option.

Juvenile Myoclonic Epilepsy

Juvenile myoclonic epilepsy is the most common adolescent- and young adult–onset GE syndrome, causing 5–10% of all cases of epilepsy (up to 18% of GEs); it has a prevalence of 1–3 in 10,000 of the general population.[2] Typical age of onset is 10–24 years, with a slightly higher ratio of females to males affected, although the range can be 8–40 years (Figure 3.1). Up to 15% of patients with JME had CAE.

The most common seizure type is myoclonic jerks that are associated with an ictal generalized polyspike-and-wave discharge. Generalized tonic–clonic seizures (GTCs) are seen in more than 90% of patients with JME and often occur upon waking or after sleep deprivation.[2] Absence seizures occur in approximately one-third of patients and are relatively brief

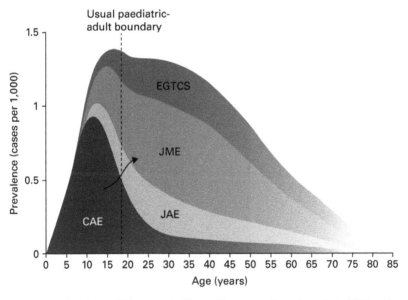

FIGURE 3.1 Prevalence of GEs across the lifespan. The arrow reflects that patients initially with CAE can transition to have other types of epilepsy, including JME, as they age. CAE, childhood absence epilepsy; EGTCS, epilepsy with generalized tonic–clonic seizures alone; JAE, juvenile absence epilepsy; JME, juvenile myoclonic epilepsy. Image from Vorderwülbecke et al.[3]

(<10 seconds in duration). Most patients will have a normal neurological exam, including normal intelligence; if mild intellectual disability is present, chromosomal microarray testing should be undertaken because microdeletions can be found in up to 10% of patients. Patients with JME may have increased frontal lobe dysfunction, which can present with increased risk-taking behaviors or drug abuse.

Interictal EEG shows irregular, generalized fast polyspike-wave and spike-wave discharges at 4–6 Hz in both wakefulness and sleep. Sleep deprivation and photic stimulation can help bring out epileptiform discharges; hyperventilation can rarely trigger seizures.

Valproic acid is the medication of choice for JME because it provides the highest rate of seizure control (up to 85% have seizure freedom), although as discussed above, it is not the preferred option for people of childbearing potential (Figure 3.2). Lamotrigine and levetiracetam are good alternatives in this patient population.

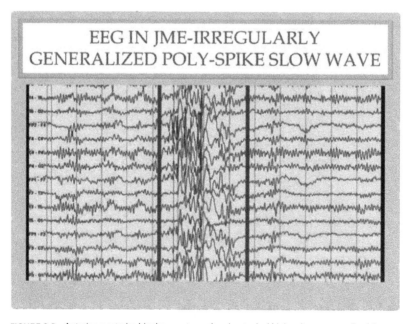

FIGURE 3.2 Anterior–posterior bipolar montage showing typical high-voltage generalized 3- or 4-Hz spike polyspike wave characteristic for JME.

Childhood and Juvenile Absence Epilepsy

Childhood absence epilepsy typically occurs in 4- to 13-year-olds and presents with typical starring spells (absence seizures) that last on average 3–20 seconds.[2] Seizures may occur daily or multiple times per day and can be triggered by hyperventilation. Even without EEG, a common practice in pediatric neurology clinics is to screen for absence epilepsy with hyperventilation, which can assist in diagnosis and the evaluation of treatment response. Oral or manual automatisms may occur in 86% of patients, and eye involvement may occur in 76.5% of children.[2]

Typical interictal EEG patterns include typical 2.5- to 4-Hz generalized spike-and-wave discharges, polyspike and wave in drowsiness or sleep, and occipital intermittent rhythmic delta activity. Photic stimulation may trigger spike-and-wave discharges but does not typically induce seizures. Ictal EEGs show 2.5- to 4-Hz generalized spike-and-wave discharges with associated absence seizure if the discharges persist for longer than 3 seconds. This typical 3-Hz generalized spike-and-wave differs from the fast 4- to 6-Hz polyspike and spike-and-wave discharges seen in JME. In addition, this threshold of 3 seconds of discharges to define an electroclinical seizure differs from the traditional threshold of an electrographic seizure being at least 10 seconds long because of empiric evidence that when patients are tested, clinically apparent lapse of awareness occurs in greater than 95% of patients with typical 3-Hz generalized spike-and-wave lasting longer than 3 seconds.

Workup otherwise involves a good history with semiology of the event and a routine 20- to 30-minute EEG with hyperventilation; if there are no ictal discharges with hyperventilation, CAE can effectively be ruled out. CAE often resolves by early adolescence in approximately 60% of patients; in the remaining patients, it may evolve into a different type of GE.[2] If absence seizures begin prior to age 4 years, or if the patient has intellectual disability or concurrent movement disorders, genetic testing for SLC2A1 testing should occur.

In childhood, ethosuximide if often the first-line treatment. Lamotrigine and valproic acid are also considered first-line treatments, but valproic acid is associated with a higher rate of side effects. Second-line treatments include levetiracetam, benzodiazepines such as clobazam, zonisamide, and topiramate. During pregnancy, lamotrigine, levetiracetam, and zonisamide are preferred options.

JAE has a similar seizure semiology to CAE except that it typically starts later than CAE (age of onset between ages 8 and 20 years; normal onset between ages 8 and 13 years). Absence seizures occur less frequently per day than in CAE, and more than 90% of JAE patients also have comorbid GTCs.[2] Patients with JAE are more likely to have attention-deficit/hyperactivity disorder and learning problems, as well as higher rates of depression and anxiety, compared to the general population. EEG demonstrates paroxysmal 3- to 5.5-Hz generalized spike-and-wave discharges that can fragment during sleep and are diagnostic during a starring spell for absence seizure. Patients with JAE are more likely to require lifelong ASM treatment. Given the high rate of comorbid GTCs, monotherapy with an ASM that treats generalized epilepsy is preferred as the first-line treatment option (Table 3.1). Fast-inactivation sodium channel agents should be avoided because they can potentially worsen seizures and precipitate absence status epilepticus (e.g., carbamazepine, oxcarbazepine, or phenytoin). Absence status epilepticus is defined as an absence seizure lasting longer than 10 continuous minutes, and it typically lasts 3 or 4 hours.

Epilepsy With Generalized Tonic–Clonic Seizures Alone

Epilepsy with generalized tonic–clonic seizures alone (EGTCS) is a common type of GE that presents with GTCs in late adolescence through young adulthood (10–25 years on average; range: 5–40 years).[2] GTCs are infrequent (sometimes less than once per year) and often require lifelong treatment, although some patients choose not to treat with daily ASMs given the rarity of their seizures. Sleep deprivation, fatigue. and alcohol are common triggers. EEG shows generalized spike-and-wave or polyspike-and-wave discharges at 3–5.5 Hz. Epileptiform discharges may be provoked by photic stimulation but are best seen during sleep deprivation or sleep.[2] Treatment with an ASM for GE is usually effective, with preference for levetiracetam or lamotrigine for people planning pregnancy in the near future (see Table 3.1).

Eyelid Myoclonia With Absences

Eyelid myoclonia with absences (EMA; previously called Jeavons syndrome) accounts for approximately 7% of all GEs.[6] The average age at onset is 5–10 years, and only a minority of patients (approximately one-third)

TABLE 3.1 Antiseizure Medication Treatments for Generalized Epilepsies

GE Syndrome	First-Line ASMs	Second-Line ASMs	Preferred in Pregnancy
JME	VPA	LTG, LEV, CLB, TPM, ZNS, BRI, LAC	LTG, LEV, ZNS
CAE	SUX, LTG, VPA	LEV, ZNS, CLB, ZNS, TPM, BRI, LAC	LTG > LEV, ZNS
JAE	VPA, LEV, LTG, ZNS, TPM	CLB, BRI, LAC	LTG, LEV, ZNS
EGTCS	VPA, LEV, LTG, ZNS, TPM	CLB, BRI, LAC	LTG or LEV > ZNS
EMA	Combinations of VPA, LEV, LTG, ZNS, TPM	CLB, BRI	LTG ± LEV < ZNS

ASM, antiseizure medication; BRI, brivaracetam; CAE, childhood absence epilepsy; CLB, clobazam; EGTCS, epilepsy with generalized tonic–clonic seizures alone; EMA, eyelid myoclonia with absences; GE, generalized epilepsy; JAE, juvenile absence epilepsy; JME, juvenile myoclonic epilepsy; LAC, lacosamide; LEV, levetiracetam; LTG, lamotrigine; SUX, ethosuximide; TPM, topiramate; VPA, valproic acid; ZNS, zonisamide.

will have remission of seizures during their lifetime.[7] A recent cohort study noted that there appeared to be two clusters of EMA: Cluster 1 comprised patients with eyelid myoclonia only and had a high likelihood of seizure remission; cluster 2 included patients with early age of onset of seizures, higher rate of intellectual disability, EEG showing generalized paroxysmal fast activity, a history of febrile seizures or status epilepticus, and often a poor response to ASMs.[7]

EMA presents with eyelid myoclonia with or without associated absence seizures, eye closure–induced generalized EEG paroxysms, and photosensitivity. The EEG in EMA is characterized by 3- to 6-Hz spike/polyspike and wave discharges associated with eyelid myoclonia. Triggers include hyperventilation, photic stimulation, and near universal seizure with eye closure in the presence of light.[6]

Combinations of ASMs typically used for treatment of GEs (see Table 3.1) are often prescribed. EMA that persists into adulthood is frequently treatment-resistant. Fast-inactivation sodium channel agents, including oxcarbazepine, carbamazepine, eslicarbazepine, and phenytoin, should be avoided because they can worsen seizures. Nonmedication options include blue lens glasses and adoption of the ketogenic or modified Atkins diet. For people with EMA who present to the neurology clinic and desire pregnancy, levetiracetam, lamotrigine, or both are often recommended in combination with the above nonmedication options.

SELECTION AND MANAGEMENT OF ASMS

The woman discussed in this case has JME. Given her young age and female sex, there are several potential considerations to discuss when choosing an ASM: the effect of an ASM on her other medical conditions, potential medication interactions including with birth control, long-term side effects, and teratogenic risk during a potential pregnancy. In the context of this patient, there are several potentially efficacious medications.

As discussed previously, valproic acid is one of the most common ASMs used in people with JME. There are, however, considerable data documenting the teratogenic side effects of valproic acid, as well as long-term negative effects on fetal cognitive development (fetal valproate syndrome)[8] and an untoward side effect profile (polycystic ovarian syndrome, weight gain, and menstrual cycle irregularities). Therefore, despite its efficacy, it may not be the first choice of medication for people with JME planning to carry a pregnancy.

Levetiracetam with or without the addition of lamotrigine is the first-choice option for people with childbearing potential and comorbid GEs planning pregnancy or at high risk for an unplanned pregnancy. Other options for GE include brivaracetam, clobazam, zonisamide, topiramate, and lacosamide, but these either do not have enough data to accurately state safety or have been associated with an increased risk of congenital malformations over lamotrigine and levetiracetam.[9] Monotherapy at the lowest doses possible is the desired option, although polytherapy may be required in some cases because breakthrough seizures during pregnancy can harm the mother and fetus. The choice of hormonal birth control or hormone treatment and its interactions is discussed further in Chapter 5B.

Potentially due to the epilepsy (and not the ASMs), people with epilepsy have approximately twice the risk of neural tube defects (NTDs). Maternal folate deficiency has been linked with the development of NTDs, and periconceptional folate supplementation has been associated with a reduction of risk. The current recommendation is 1 mg of folate for all people with epilepsy of childbearing potential given a recent study showing a potential for cancer risk at higher doses.[10] There has been substantial controversy regarding this finding, and therefore further study is needed.

A prepregnancy ASM level should be obtained, and monthly ASM levels should be checked throughout the pregnancy to target the prepregnancy level or slightly higher. In some studies, ASM levels less than 65% of prepregnancy baseline were associated with increased worsening of seizures. This is especially true of the following ASMs: levetiracetam, lamotrigine, zonisamide, and oxcarbazepine. ASM levels may drop in the first and second trimester due to increased clearance and physiologic blood volume in the mother, triggering an unintended breakthrough seizure. For certain medications, this increased clearance may occur prior to the person knowing that they are pregnant. In addition, the serum level of certain medications may fluctuate substantially over the course of the day (e.g., levetiracetam). Therefore, it is important for the ASM level to be obtained at the same time relative to the last dose so that these levels are comparable throughout the peripartum period (as discussed further in Chapter 5B).

There are not special considerations for mode of delivery in people with epilepsy. ASMs should be taken as scheduled, irrespective of oral intake status. Levels may need to be adjusted postpartum as the mother's renal clearance returns to baseline levels. Pre-existing epilepsy or non-eclamptic seizures are not an indication to have cesarean section or induction of labor. The literature has shown that at sites without access to high-risk obstetric care, there was an increased rate of cesarean section, which may expose patients to unnecessary surgical risk. Patients who are in status epilepticus may require a cesarean section if there is a threat to the life of mother and fetus; this is discussed further in Chapter 6.

In this case, after a discussion with the patient about the risks and benefits of each ASM, she opted to start levetiracetam. She achieved good control of her seizures; however, her anxiety worsened, so lamotrigine was gradually titrated up and levetiracetam withdrawn. Folate supplementation (1 mg) was begun at the time of ASM initiation. She was educated about the role of sleep deprivation as an epilepsy trigger, instructed as to safety concerns, and told not to drive for 6 months from the date of her last seizure.

KEY POINTS TO REMEMBER

- Valproic acid is the most effective ASM for GEs in general, but due to concerns about teratogenicity, other ASMs (levetiracetam, lamotrigine, zonisamide, and brivaracetam) may be better options for people with childbearing potential.
- ASM decisions should be based on discussion between the patient and provider that includes information about potential safety issues during pregnancy and potential interactions with birth control/hormonal therapy.
- Prepregnancy ASM level(s) should be obtained, and ASM levels should be checked monthly during pregnancy to prevent a breakthrough seizure from drug levels dropping.
- People with epilepsy in the childbearing years on an ASM should also be taking folate supplementation (ideally 1 mg daily).

References

1. Geurrini R, Marini C, Mantegazza M. Genetic epilepsy syndromes without structural brain abnormalities: Clinical features and experimental models. *Neurotherapeutics*. 2014;11(2):269–285.
2. Hirsch E, French J, Scheffer IE, et al. ILAE definition of the idiopathic generalized epilepsy syndromes: Position statement by the ILAE Task Force on Nosology and Definitions. *Epilepsia*. 2022;63(6):1475–1499.
3. Vorderwülbecke BJ, Wandschneider B, Weber Y, Holtkamp M. Genetic generalized epilepsies in adults: Challenging assumptions and dogmas. *Nat Rev Neurol*. 2022;18:71–83.
4. Serafini A, Gerard E, Genton P, Crespel A, Gelisse P. Treatment of juvenile myoclonic epilepsy in patients of child-bearing potential. *CNS Drugs*. 2019;33:195–208.
5. Bui, E. Women's issues in epilepsy. *Epilepsy*. 2022;28(2):399–427.
6. Joshi CN, Patrick J. Eyelid myoclonia with absences: Routine EEG is sufficient to make a diagnosis. *Seizure*. 2007;16(3):254–260.

7. Cerulli Irelli E, Cocchi E, Ramantani G, et al. Electroclinical features and long-term seizure outcome in patients with eyelid myoclonia with absences. *Neurology.* 2022;98(18):e1865–e1876.
8. Cohen JM, Alvestad S, Cesta CE, et al. Comparative safety of antiseizure medication monotherapy for major malformations. *Ann Neurol.* 2023; 93(3):551–562.
9. McCluskey G, Kinney MO, Russell A, et al. Zonisamide safety in pregnancy: Data from the UK and Ireland epilepsy and pregnancy register. *Seizure.* 2021;91:311–315.
10. Vegrim HM, Dreier JW, Alvestad S, et al. Cancer risk in children of mothers with epilepsy and high-dose folic acid use in pregnancy. *JAMA Neurol.* 2022;79(11):1130–1138.

4 Functional Neurologic Symptoms

Emily L. Johnson

A 24-year-old woman is referred for evaluation of recent onset of episodes of behavior arrest, inability to speak, and bilateral irregular arm movements that intermittently come and go. These episodes last 20–30 minutes, and during the episodes she may also have lacrimation. Afterwards, she reports that she can remember the episodes and can hear people talking to her but cannot speak or control her movements during the episodes. She has had a brain MRI and routine electroencephalogram (EEG), which were normal. Her only medication is escitalopram for depression.

She is admitted for inpatient video-EEG monitoring, which records two typical episodes of inability to speak or control movements. EEG is normal throughout these episodes.

What do you do now?

FUNCTIONAL NEUROLOGIC DISORDERS

Functional neurologic disorder (FND) is an umbrella term covering neurologic symptoms manifesting in various ways, with the commonality that no underlying organic cause is present as an explanation for the symptoms. Symptoms can involve motor, sensory, speech, or a combination of functions, and they can be fixed or paroxysmal. FND are relatively common, with an incidence of 4–12 per 100,000 annually.[1] Previous terminology, such as conversion disorder and pseudoseizures, is no longer preferred in favor of FND. FND is distinguished from voluntarily produced symptoms (factitious disorder and malingering).

Evaluation and Diagnosis of FND

Evaluation depends on a thorough examination and review of the patient's history. If symptoms are paroxysmal, supportive history from people who have witnessed an event or video of an event is paramount. For suspected non-epileptic seizures (NES), the gold standard is video-EEG with recording of a typical event to correlate symptoms with simultaneous electrocerebral activity. Normal EEG during bilateral motor symptoms or unresponsiveness is diagnostic of NES. However, certain symptoms, such as eye closure during episodes, stopping/starting movements that are not rhythmic, irregular movements, and pelvic thrusting, are supportive of NES rather than epileptic seizure (Table 4.1).

Physical examination during functional motor symptoms (tremor and weakness) can identify signs suggestive of FND, including an entrainable tremor (e.g., a tremor that changes frequency to match movement of the contralateral limb or other task set by the examiner) or distractibility.[2] The Hoover sign is an examination maneuver by which strength of an affected limb is indirectly tested: In the case of right leg weakness, for example, a seated patient may be unable to provide downward pressure when the right leg is directly tested. However, when the examiner instructs the patient to raise the unaffected left leg, while the examiner places a hand under the affected right knee, the patient may involuntarily produce downward pressure with the right leg while exerting effort to elevate the left leg.

TABLE 4.1 **Features Suggestive of Functional Neurologic Disorder (FND) Episodes versus Epileptic Seizures (ES)**

Sign	Odds Ratio of association with FND versus ES
Fluctuating course	OR 37.37 (95% CI 13.56–102.96, p < 0.001)[1]
Head shaking	OR 2.95 (95% CI 1.26–6.79, p = 0.012)[1]
Hip thrusting	OR 4.28 (95% CI 1.21–15.18, p = 0.02)[1]
Longer duration	OR 2.26 (95% CI 1.15–4.45, p = 0.018)[2]
Automatisms	OR 0.05 (95% CI 0.004–0.634, p = 0.021)[2]

[1]Duncan AJ, Peric I, Boston R, Seneviratne U. Predictive semiology of psychogenic non-epileptic seizures in an epilepsy monitoring unit. *J Neurol.* 2022 Apr;269(4):2172–2178. doi:10.1007/s00415-021-10805-1. Epub 2021 Sep 22. PMID: 34550469; PMCID: PMC8456070.
[2]Lombardi N, Scévola L, Sarudiansky M, Giagante B, Gargiulo A, Alonso N, Stivala EG, Oddo S, Fernandez-Lima M, Kochen S, Guido Korman, D'Alessio L. Differential semiology based on video electroencephalography monitoring between psychogenic nonepileptic seizures and temporal lobe epileptic seizures. *J Acad Consult Liaison Psychiatry.* 2021 Jan-Feb;62(1):22–28. doi:10.1016/j.psym.2020.07.003. Epub 2020 Jul 22. PMID: 32950266.

Sensory symptoms that split exactly at the midline are suggestive of FND. In cases of functional vision loss, presenting strong stimuli to the patient such as a tilting mirror can elicit tracking.

Extremely effortful speech, prosodic abnormalities ("foreign accent syndrome"), and dysfluency with inconsistent stuttering in the absence of vocal cord or neurologic pathology are manifestations of speech-related FND. Distractibility and inconsistency throughout the examination are suggestive of FND.

Risk Factors and Basis for FND

Traditionally, FND has been thought of as a manifestation of psychological distress. Patients with FND are more likely to have a history of sexual or physical abuse than are patients without FND, and women (particularly young women) are overrepresented. Other triggers or commonalities, such as chronic or acute pain and psychiatric comorbidities, are common. More recently, research has focused on identifying how symptoms are produced through neurobiological means. Attentional dysregulation, in which there is a mismatch between "bottom-up sensory information" and "top-down predictions about the nature of the expected sensory information," is one area of investigation.[1] Functional neuroimaging has revealed alterations in supplementary motor area activation, decreased supplementary motor area and limbic area connectivity, and abnormally increased connectivity between emotional regulation areas and executive function. Notably, these alterations in connectivity are not present when patients are instructed to deliberately produce symptoms (i.e., as in malingering).

Treatment of FND

Discussing the diagnosis with the patient is a critical part of treatment for FND. The patient with FND should not come away with the impression that the neurologist thinks "it's all in your head." Presenting the diagnosis in a nonjudgmental way, conveying the certainty and support for the diagnosis of FND, and discussing the treatability of FND are key to patient acceptance (which in turn is key to treatment success).

Psychological interventions are the mainstay of treatment for patients with FND.[3] Structured, disorder-adapted cognitive–behavioral therapy is the treatment of choice for NES and functional movement disorders in particular. Physical therapy is also recognized as an important part of multidisciplinary treatment, with a focus on rehabilitation of normal control of movements or speech. If the FND patient has comorbid anxiety or depression, these should also be treated appropriately with anxiolytics, antidepressants, and targeted therapy. Neurologic agents in patients without neurologic disease should be avoided due to inefficacy and risk of side effects (e.g., antiseizure medications should not be used to treat NES).

KEY POINTS TO REMEMBER

- FND are relatively common.
- FND are distinct from voluntary or manufactured symptoms (factitious disorder, malingering, and confabulating).
- Treatment involves validation of the patient's symptoms and acceptance of the diagnosis, along with targeted cognitive–behavioral therapy, physical therapy, and treatment of psychiatric comorbidities as needed.

References

1. Espay AJ, Aybek S, Carson A, et al. Current concepts in diagnosis and treatment of functional neurological disorders. *JAMA Neurol*. 2018;75(9):1132–1141. doi:10.1001/jamaneurol.2018.1264
2. Patwal R, Jolly AJ, Kumar A, Yadav R, Desai G, Thippeswamy H. Diagnostic accuracy of clinical signs and investigations for functional weakness, sensory and movement disorders: A systematic review. *J Psychosom Res*. 2023;168:111196. doi:10.1016/j.jpsychores.2023.111196
3. LaFrance WC Jr, Baird GL, Barry JJ, et al; NES Treatment Trial (NEST-T) Consortium. Multicenter pilot treatment trial for psychogenic nonepileptic seizures: A randomized clinical trial. *JAMA Psychiatry*. 2014;71(9):997–1005. doi:10.1001/jamapsychiatry.2014.817

5A A Young Woman With Epilepsy and PCOS

M. Angela O'Neal, Revised by Caroline Just, Ginette Moores, and Esther Bui

A 24-year-old woman with epilepsy presents to your clinic. Her seizures began at age 12 years. She experiences no aura; witnesses report behavioural arrest, then tonic and clonic movements with associated incontinence. She experiences 30 minutes of postictal confusion. Prior brain MRI was normal, and previous electroencephalograms have demonstrated a left temporal epileptiform focus. Since age 15 years, she has been on valproate, with no seizures for 2 years.

In that time she gained 30 lbs. She weighs 225 lbs at 64 inches tall, with central adiposity and male pattern alopecia. She has irregular periods for which she was recently evaluated by a gynecologist. Her labs showed an elevated testosterone level, and imaging showed multiple ovarian cysts. A diagnosis of polycystic ovarian syndrome (PCOS) was made.

Her medications are a Mirena intrauterine device and Depakote ER 750 mg bid.

What do you do now?

THE RELATIONSHIP BETWEEN HORMONES AND SEIZURES

Progesterone is generally anticonvulsive, and estrogen is generally proconvulsive. There are numerous reports that epilepsy, particularly focal epilepsy, can cause hypothalamic dysfunction. However, many of these studies are confounded by being retrospective, using subjects who presented to tertiary epilepsy centers and concurrently taking antiseizure medications (ASMs). There are multiple connections between the limbic cortex and hypothalamus that modulate the hypothalamus–pituitary hormonal secretion. For example, following a generalized seizure, prolactin levels can increase by three- or fourfold. Gonadotropin-releasing hormone (GnRH) levels may also be altered following seizures. Altered GnRH may lead to abnormal release of follicle-stimulating hormone and luteinizing hormone, with downstream direct effects on ovulation and the maturation of ovarian follicles. Although it was previously thought that women with epilepsy (WWE) had reduced fertility compared to controls, a 2018 cohort study determined no difference in time to conception or fertility compared to controls.[1]

Antiseizure Drugs and Polycystic Ovarian Syndrome

Valproate is the ASM most associated with PCOS. PCOS is a diagnosis made on ultrasound and per anatomical criteria, with these showing the presence of multiple ovarian cysts. The National Institutes of Health consensus definition of PCOS includes the presence of menstrual dysfunction; clinical evidence of hyperandrogenism; and exclusion of other endocrinopathies, such as Cushing syndrome and hypothyroidism. Valproate can directly increase ovarian testosterone production. It can also cause weight gain, leading to insulin resistance, another mechanism contributing to PCOS. One study examined switching women with PCOS from valproate to lamotrigine. In the subsequent year, the women had significant weight loss, decreased androgen levels, and a decrease in the number of ovarian follicles.[2]

In our patient, the significant weight gain of 30 pounds may be related to valproate, thus contributing to the metabolic syndrome of PCOS. There should be consideration of switching her to another ASM, especially because there are additional teratogenic concerns in a woman of childbearing age. Levetiracetam and lamotrigine would be good choices as an ASM for this woman, given its lack of hormonal effects.

KEY POINTS TO REMEMBER

- Hormones play a role in epilepsy and in ASMs.
- WWE, especially if treated with valproate, are at high risk to develop PCOS.
- PCOS is a complex disorder with both genetic and environmental contributors. It develops in women in whom the ovaries are stimulated to produce excessive testosterone.
- Prevention: Consider modification of ASM of choice in reproductive-aged women.

References

1. Pennell PB, French JA, Harden CL, Davis A, Bagiella E, Andreopoulos E, Lau C, Llewellyn N, Barnard S, Allien S. Fertility and birth outcomes in women with epilepsy seeking pregnancy. *JAMA Neurol.* 2018 Aug 1;75(8):962–969. doi:10.1001/jamaneurol.2018.0646. PMID: 29710218; PMCID: PMC6142930.
2. Bilo L, Meo R. Polycystic ovary syndrome in women using valproate: A review. *Gynecol Endocrinol.* 2008;24(10):562–570.

5B A Young Woman With Epilepsy and Family Planning

M. Angela O'Neal, Revised by Caroline Just, Ginette Moores, and Esther Bui

The patient returns for annual follow-up, now on lamotrigine 75 bid. Her last seizure was 10 months ago, due to medication noncompliance and dehydration. A drug level of 10 µg/ml (range: 3–14 µg/ml) was obtained 6 months ago. Stopping valproate led to a 25-pound weight loss and more regular menses. No changes in her seizure frequency, duration, or semiology.

Today, you obtain a detailed reproductive history. She identifies as a woman (she/her) and past sexual partners have been male and female. She and her long-term female partner hope to conceive via assisted reproductive technology (ART). She had one miscarriage (at 8 weeks), one therapeutic abortion (at 4 weeks), and no children. She currently does not use contraception but has used oral contraceptives and condoms in the past. Current medications include a daily vitamin B12 supplement, folic acid 1 mg daily, and lamotrigine 75 mg bid.

What do you do now?

PREGNANCY, ASM CHOICE, ROLE OF ART, AND TERATOGENICITY RISK FACTORS

Epilepsy is the third most common chronic neurological disorder world-wide. Unfortunately, many therapies used to treat seizure are associated with some level of risk to the fetus in utero. In 2014, the U.S. Food and Drug Administration published the "Pregnancy and Lactation Labeling Rule," which changes the format of prescription drug packaging inserts. Specifically, in the pregnancy subsection, former A, B, C, D, and X lettering categories used to designate pregnancy risk were replaced with information including a summary of risks, available data, and clinical considerations. These changes aim to better assist providers with evaluating risks versus benefits for using medications in pregnant or nursing mothers.[1]

Some ASMs have very high risks for major congenital malformations (MCMs), whereas others have only a slightly increased risk above base-line.[2] Lamotrigine and levetiracetam both had MCM rates of only 1.9%, compared to controls at 1%. Oxcarbazepine had an MCM rate of 1.6%. Valproate and topiramate had higher rates of 9.2% and 4.8%, respectively. It is also notable that the actual seizure event has been reported to increase fetal morbidity and risk pregnancy maintenance. These risks include fetal trauma related to falls, fetal heart rate deceleration, placental abruption, miscarriage, preterm labor, and premature birth.[3]

In the United States, approximately 50% of pregnancies are unplanned. In a recently reported retrospective study of 115 women on teratogenic medications, approximately 70% were not using concurrent medical con-traception. For women using contraception, oral contraceptives were the method of choice. Notably, less than 7% reported receiving any counseling for a contraceptive plan.[4,6]

A discussion about future pregnancy planning is appropriate at the first visit and at several points throughout the physician–patient relation-ship to cover treatment regimens and potential associated risks specific to a woman's life stage. There are specific concerns in that enzyme-inducing antiseizure drugs such as phenytoin, phenobarbital, and carbamazepine can reduce the efficacy of the oral contraceptive pill (OCP) by lowering serum estrogen levels. In addition, the estrogen component of the OCP can lower the serum concentration of lamotrigine, increasing the risk of seizures.[6]

Folic acid supplementation is recommended for all women of childbearing potential. Folic acid supplementation prior to pregnancy has been shown to significantly reduce the risk for neural tube defects, but more than 1 g/day may increase cancer risk in the fetus.[7] Once women begin to consider trying to conceive, they may inquire about their chances of becoming pregnant in the context of their epilepsy. WWE have had historically lower birth rates than women without epilepsy, possibly due to sociodemographic factors such as education status, employment status, and marriage status. A 2018 observation cohort study of 197 WWE seeking pregnancy showed no difference in likelihood of achieving pregnancy, time to pregnancy, and live birth rates compared with their peers without epilepsy.[8]

For WWE facing fertility challenges, ART is increasingly being used to achieve pregnancy in the setting of infertility, among single or LGBTQ+ patients, for those who require preimplantation genetic testing, and for fertility preservation. Often, this involves hormonal manipulation to increase the chances of attaining pregnancy. Although two previous case reports have raised concern for seizure worsening following ART, a more recent retrospective chart review of 12 WWE who underwent ART did not identify any exacerbation of seizures. Reassuringly, in a population-based cohort, WWE taking ASMs were as likely to have a liveborn child after ART compared to women without epilepsy and WWE not on ASMs. Although further research in this area is needed, the studies thus far are reassuring that ART is effective and may be safely performed in WWE.[9]

Once a pregnancy has been confirmed, it is important to link the patient with the appropriate obstetric providers to best evaluate the fetus over the course of the pregnancy, as well as offer more education to the parents. If the patient is on a teratogenic agent, considering the patient's wishes to continue or terminate the pregnancy might also present a need for referral to outside appropriate providers.

Up to 50% of pregnancies in the United States are unplanned, with this rate similarly observed among WWE. This is important to remember when treating this population, who are on continuous treatment with known teratogens. Organogenesis occurs within the first 4–10 weeks of gestation (postconception), and structural abnormalities established during this window will be irreversible. Therefore, pregnancy planning should be a topic of discussion for any WWE of childbearing age, ideally prior to pregnancy. However, beyond the first trimester, ASM exposure, particularly valproate, in the second and third trimesters may impact early childhood neurodevelopment. Research is ongoing to fully understand the neurodevelopmental outcomes of in utero ASM exposure, led by the Maternal Outcomes and Neurodevelopmental Effects of Antiepileptic Drugs study in the United States.

For preconception planning, folic acid supplementation should be initiated, and the ASM dose should be reviewed to determine the lowest effective dose. Considerations can also be made to transition, if safely possible, to alternate ASMs with lower teratogenicity rates, such as levetiracetam, lamotrigine, and oxcarbazepine.

> The patient continues on her lamotrigine 75 bid with folic acid 1 mg daily and successfully conceives through ART (in utero insemination). At 14 weeks of gestation, she presents to the emergency room with a breakthrough convulsive seizure. She reports good compliance, but her lamotrigine level is undetectable.

During pregnancy, metabolism of ASMs changes significantly. For lamotrigine, clearance can increase from 65% to 230% due to induction of glucuronidation by estrogen. Even two different pregnancies in the same patient can result in different increases in lamotrigine clearance. In the case of levetiracetam, levels are affected by increased renal clearance in pregnancy. Average peak clearance increased by 207%.[9] It is thus important to monitor levels of these medications throughout pregnancy (monthly) and increase the dose accordingly. For lamotrigine, it is similarly important to reduce the dose shortly before delivery to avoid toxicity.

> The patient's lamotrigine is increased slowly to 150 bid in the second trimester and 250 bid in the third trimester, maintaining a level of 8 or 9 µg/ml, monitored monthly by her neurologist. She delivers a healthy baby boy via vaginal delivery. On postpartum

day 3, she begins a prescheduled lamotrigine taper from 250 mg bid slowly over 4 weeks to 150 mg bid. At her 1-month postpartum visit, she is doing well and remains seizure-free. She agrees to lower her lamotrigine down to her prepregnancy dose of 100 mg bid and achieves this dose over a 2-week taper schedule. At 12 months postpartum, she returns with a healthy, normally developing infant and speaks to you about planning her second pregnancy.

KEY POINTS TO REMEMBER

- Prevention: Frequently discuss pregnancy planning, pregnancy prevention, and common drug–drug interactions in all patients on therapy.
- Prevention: Folic acid supplementation prior to pregnancy has been shown to significantly reduce the risk for neural tube defects, but more than 1 g/day may increase cancer risk in the fetus.
- Evaluation: Always order a pregnancy test for patients with reasonable risk factors prior to prescribing high-risk teratogenic therapies.
- Ethics and referral: Make referral for fertility and reproductive health assessment and education for patients.
- Pharmacokinetics knowledge is crucial for managing WWE during pregnancy, and levels need to be checked frequently for most ASMs.
- Practice advice: (1) Lowest ASM dose possible; (2) individualized target ASM levels, slightly higher than preconception levels; and (3) regular ASM level checks during pregnancy.

References

1. U.S. Food and Drug Administration. Pregnancy and lactation labeling (drugs) final rule. 2014. Accessed May 30, 2023. http://www.fda.gov/Drugs/Development ApprovalProcess/DevelopmentResources/Labeling/ucm093307.htm

2. The North American AED Pregnancy Registry. Annual update for 2022. 2022. Accessed May 30, 2023. https://www.aedpregnancyregistry.org/annual-upd ate-for-2022

3. Kaplan PW, Norwitz ER, Ben-Menachem E, et al. Obstetric risks for women with epilepsy during pregnancy. *Epilepsy Behav*. 2007;11(3):283–291.

4. Bhakta J, Bainbridge J, Borgelt L. Teratogenic medications and concurrent contraceptive use and women of childbearing ability with epilepsy. *Epilepsy Behav*. 2015;52(Pt A):212–217.

5. Borgelt LM, Hart FM, Bainbridge JL. Epilepsy during pregnancy: Focus on management strategies. *Int J Womens Health*. 2016;8:505–517.

6. Reimers A, Brodtkorb E, Sabers A. Interactions between hormonal contraception and antiepileptic drugs: Clinical and mechanistic considerations. *Seizure*. 2015;28:66–70.

7. Vegrim HM, Dreier JW, Alvestad S, et al. Cancer risk in children of mothers with epilepsy and high-dose folic acid use during pregnancy. *JAMA Neurol*. 2022;79(11):1130–1138. doi:10.1001/jamaneurol.2022.2977

8. Pennell PB, French JA, Harden CL, et al. Fertility and birth outcomes in women with epilepsy seeking pregnancy. *JAMA Neurol*. 2018;75(8):962–969.

9. Bui E. Women's issues in epilepsy. *Continuum*. 2022;28(2):399–427.

6 Frequent Seizures During Pregnancy

Christina R. Catherine and

Alexandra Urban

A 28-year-old woman who is 34 weeks pregnant presents to the emergency department via ambulance after her husband witnessed two generalized tonic–clonic (GTC) seizures without return to baseline. She has epilepsy and takes levetiracetam and clonazepam. The husband reports no recent infections, fevers/chills, or missed doses of antiseizure medication. The patient received one dose of midazolam intramuscularly en route. She is somnolent with no clear focal deficits on examination. Vitals show heart rate 125 beats per minute and blood pressure 120/67 mmHg. The initial investigations are unremarkable (complete blood counts, basic metabolic panel, and urine protein/creatinine ratio). An additional GTC is witnessed prior to the brain MRI.

What do you do now?

STATUS EPILEPTICUS DURING PREGNANCY

Status epilepticus (SE) during pregnancy is a medical emergency. Immediate treatment with benzodiazepines should be initiated. The first-line antiseizure medication (ASM) in pregnancy is levetiracetam, and it should be co-administered with benzodiazepine treatment. Phenytoin can also be considered but does have additional significant potential side effects in the mother and fetus. For the fetus, these include cleft palate, vitamin K and D deficiency, and potential for cardiac and limb malformations. Mothers are at a potentially increased risk for postpartum hemorrhage. Newer ASMs, such as lacosamide and brivaracetam, are other options with minimal safety data during pregnancy and the early postpartum period. Treatment with intravenous (IV) magnesium should be initiated if there is concern for eclampsia. Prior to the MagPIE trial, the use of other ASMs (diazepam and phenytoin) in patients with eclampsia was sometimes undertaken. Postpartum eclampsia or ongoing seizures despite IV magnesium usage may necessitate the use of other ASMs such as levetiracetam until other causes of new-onset seizures are ruled out. Neuroimaging is necessary and prioritized based on suspected etiology; either computed tomography with appropriate shielding of the fetus or magnetic resonance imaging to determine a potential structural cause of seizures should be urgently undertaken. Magnetic resonance angiography without contrast can safely be performed in pregnancy if there is concern for a vascular cause of symptoms. Initial blood work includes complete blood count, basic metabolic panel, liver function testing, urine protein:creatinine ratio, urine drug screen, and coagulopathy testing. An urgent lumbar puncture should be pursued for concern of central nervous system (CNS) infection. The cerebrospinal fluid testing includes cell counts; glucose; protein; viral polymerase chain reactions for herpes simplex 1 and 2, cytomegalovirus, and varicella zoster virus; bacterial culture with Gram stain; and syphilis screening if appropriate. The patient should be cared for at a tertiary care facility with maternal–fetal medicine, critical care medicine, neonatology and neurology specialists.

If seizures persist despite benzodiazepine and first-line ASM treatment, standard SE guidelines apply, including intubating the patient and the use of IV anesthetics. Despite the safety of lamotrigine during pregnancy, the necessary slow up-titration curve prevents its usage in SE. Other potential

ASM options to consider beyond levetiracetam and phenytoin include oral ASMs oxcarbazepine, gabapentin, carbamazepine, and topiramate (the latter being safer in the third trimester)[1] or IV lacosamide/brivaracetam (although data are limited for these newer IV medications). Valproic acid should be avoided and administered only if all other ASMs have failed, and it is preferable that the patient not be in the first trimester.[2] During pregnancy, propofol and midazolam are preferred, but ketamine, phenobarbital, and pentobarbital have been used in various case reports.[2,3] In cases of super-refractory SE that is endangering the life of the pregnant person, termination of pregnancy via delivery or abortion is recommended but should be timed with the help of neonatology and maternal–fetal medicine.[2,3] Pregnancies between 25 and 32 weeks gestational age (GA) should be delivered following induction of lung maturity, whereas pregnancies greater than 32 weeks GA can be immediately delivered.[4]

The cause of SE should be quickly identified. There are two main groups of pregnant people who have SE during pregnancy: those with a prior history of epilepsy (as in this case) and those with new-onset status epilepticus in pregnancy.[4] In patients with epilepsy, SE is thought to be secondary to reductions in ASM levels via increased clearance or reduced adherence. New-onset SE in pregnancy is most commonly caused by eclampsia, posterior reversible encephalopathy syndrome (PRES), reversible cerebral vasoconstrictor syndrome (RCVS), or cerebral venous sinus thrombosis (CVST). Comorbid eclampsia may be present with RCVS or PRES. Less common causes of new-onset SE in pregnancy include drug abuse (cocaine, methamphetamines, and synthetic marijuana), autoimmune encephalitis, subarachnoid hemorrhage, cavernoma, brain tumor, pyridoxine deficiency, cavernoma, CNS infection, or porphyria.[3,4]

Prolonged seizure activity in the mother is associated with significant morbidity and mortality in both mother and fetus. In pregnant patients, SE can cause abnormalities in placental blood flow leading to fetal distress, fetal hypoxia, possible neurodevelopmental delay, and increased risk of preterm birth.[3] The incidence of SE ranges from 5 to 40 per 100,000 people, with an average annual incidence of 12.6 per 100,000 and even less in the pregnant population.[3] Pregnancy-related SE has been reported to occur in 0.6% of pregnancies in people with epilepsy.[5]

Outcomes for SE during pregnancy vary by study. A Danish study examining pregnancy outcomes noted that the maternal mortality rate for mothers with epilepsy was 41.7 per 100,000 pregnancies versus 8.2 per 100,000 for control pregnancies.[4] This increased maternal mortality rate for mothers was in part attributed to SE during pregnancy. A 2006 EURAP registry study of 1,956 pregnancies in 1,882 pregnant people with epilepsy (PPWE) noted that 3.5% of patients had seizures during childbirth, 2% of patients had SE, and there was one stillbirth but no maternal deaths in the SE group.[4] Maternal and fetal outcomes are generally good, with low mortality rates noted in the developed world for mothers with epilepsy complicated by SE during pregnancy.[4] This is unfortunately not always the case in the developing world, where access to appropriate care may not be easily available,[5] or in people with new-onset SE in pregnancy, where the underlying cause of SE may be the driver of maternal mortality.

KEY POINTS TO REMEMBER

- Status epilepticus in pregnancy is a medical emergency for both the mother and the fetus, with potential for high morbidity or mortality for both patients.
- Seizures should be promptly treated with a benzodiazepine and first-line ASM. The mother should be cared for at a tertiary care center with a multidisciplinary team consisting of maternal–fetal medicine, a critical care team, neonatology, and neurology.
- A cause of SE should be identified. Common causes of SE in pregnancy are missed ASM doses in PPWE, preeclampsia/eclampsia, drug abuse (cocaine, synthetic marijuana, and methamphetamines), CNS infections, brain tumor, RCVS, PRES, CVST, and stroke.
- There are currently no consensus guidelines on whether vaginal delivery at or near term should be pursued versus more immediate labor induction or cesarean section. The mode of delivery is to be determined through a multidisciplinary approach based on the status of the mother and the fetus and the gestational age of the fetus.

References

1. Putta S, Pennell PB. Management of epilepsy during pregnancy: Evidence-based strategies. *Future Neurol*. 2015;10(2):161–176. https://doi.org/10.2217/fnl.15.4

2. Roberti R, Roccas M, Iannone LF, et al. Status epilepticus in pregnancy: A literature review and a protocol proposal. *Expert Rev Neurotherapeut*. 2022;22(4):301–312. https://doi.org/10.1080/14737 175.2022.2057224

3. Carrasco C, Schwalk A, Hwang B, Iwuji K, Islam E. Super-refractory status epilepticus in a 29-year-old pregnant patient. *SAGE Open Med Case Rep*. 2021;9:2050313X211000455. doi:10.1177/2050313X211000455.

4. Rosenow F, Mann C. Status epilepticus in pregnancy. *Epilepsy Behav*. 2023;138:109034.

5. Ofeh MA, Nodem CRK. Status epilepticus and coma in pregnancy: Management dilemma in a resource limited setting: Case report. *Open J Obstet Gynecol*. 2022;12(1):25–32. doi:10.4236/ojog.2022.121003

SECTION II

Autoimmune and Paraneoplastic Disorders

7 Multiple Sclerosis

Sarah Conway and Tamara B. Kaplan

A 31-year-old woman was recently diagnosed with multiple sclerosis (MS) after she suffered from optic neuritis that completely resolved and had an MRI that fulfilled the 2024 McDonald diagnostic criteria. She would like to hold off on starting any disease-modifying therapy (DMT) until after she has a child, as she and her husband are trying to conceive. She becomes pregnant 3 months later, and her pregnancy is uneventful. She starts breastfeeding, and 1 month after delivery, she notices tingling and numbness in her lower extremities and has difficulty walking. She is treated with intravenous (IV) methylprednisolone for 5 days. She has MRIs, which show new lesions, and then is started on ocrelizumab. Two years later, she desires to get pregnant again.

What do you do now?

MULTIPLE SCLEROSIS IN PREGNANCY

Natural History

A significant number of MS patients will develop the disease during their childbearing years. Until the 1950s, women with MS were told that pregnancy could worsen their disease and were discouraged from becoming pregnant; however, based on studies during the past few decades, this information proved to be incorrect.

There was a major shift in thinking with the 1998 publication of the Pregnancy in Multiple Sclerosis (PRIMS) study, which is the best large-scale prospective study published to date. PRIMS included 254 women (246 with relapsing MS) and 269 pregnancies. Patients were followed for at least 12 months postpartum.[1]

Compared to prepregnancy, annualized relapse rate fell by 70% during the third trimester. However, during the first 3 months postpartum, the relapse rate rebounded to 70% above the prepregnancy level, but then it came down and stayed down at the prepregnancy rate after those initial 3 months. The annualized relapse rate from postpartum months 3–12 was not significantly different from that of the prepregnancy year.

A follow-up study to PRIMS examined factors that predicted a relapse and found that the risk for postpartum relapse was greatest in those who had experienced a relapse in the year prior to pregnancy or during pregnancy.[2] The findings of the PRIMS study have been replicated by numerous other studies since its initial publication. In modern cohorts, discontinuation of both natalizumab and fingolimod prior to pregnancy are risk factors for relapses during pregnancy that are often severe. Conversely, the use of B-cell-depleting agents prior to pregnancy has been associated with lower relapse rates postpartum.[3–7]

How to Treat a Relapse During Pregnancy

When there is concern for worsening disease activity during pregnancy, it is important to rule out factors that may cause "pseudo-exacerbations," such as urinary tract infections, which are more common in pregnancy.

If a relapse is severe enough to warrant therapy, most clinicians will use IV methylprednisolone. This particular corticosteroid is preferred because it is metabolized before crossing the placenta. In general, many clinicians avoid steroids during the first trimester because previous data showed a possible increased risk of cleft palate during this period. Importantly, two recent large cohort studies found no link between the use of inhaled or oral corticosteroids during the first trimester and an increased risk of cleft lip/palate or other congenital malformations in the offspring of more than 1,000 women.

Other clinicians may use IV immunoglobulin, which is thought to be safe during pregnancy and has a low rate of maternal side effects.

Avoiding Postpartum Relapses

In general, it is advised to resume immunomodulating therapy as soon as possible with DMTs that are compatible with breastfeeding. Women who defer breastfeeding can resume therapy immediately.

One study showed that monthly steroid infusions for the first 6 months postpartum seemed to reduce the relapse rate. However, there was no difference in overall neurological function or progression of disease between those treated and controls. Overall, using frequent IV steroids in the postpartum period is not the standard of care, and the use of such therapy should be on an individual basis.

Use of Disease-Modifying Therapy

In general, DMTs are not routinely continued during pregnancy. Guidelines on stopping DMT depend on which DMT the patient is on prior to conception (Table 7.1). Although there may be potential risks in conceiving while on a DMT, there may also be a risk of relapse if therapy is withheld for too long. Sphingosine-1-phosphate (S1P) receptor modulators and natalizumab have significant risk of rebound disease when stopped. For women with MS who are contemplating pregnancy, a transition to B-cell-depleting therapy is often recommended. These therapies are effective, safe to use prior to pregnancy, and can be continued postpartum given minimal transfer into breast milk.

Interferons (Rebif, Avonex, Bestaseron, and Plegridy)

Interferon-βs are the oldest class of DMTs. In primates, there appeared to be a dose–response increase in spontaneous abortions when primates were given

TABLE 7.1 **Guidelines on Stopping Disease-Modifying Therapy**

Disease-Modifying Agent	Drug Half-Life	Fetal and Maternal Risks	Pregnancy Recommendations
Interferon-β-1b and -β-1a	10 hr	Spontaneous abortions in animals; not seen in humans	Stop at positive pregnancy test; in select cases can consider continuing during pregnancy
Glatiramer acetate	1 hr	None reported	Stop at positive pregnancy test; in select cases can consider continuing during pregnancy
Fingolimod/ siponimod/ ozanimod/ ponesimod	6–9 days/ 30 hr/21 hr/ 33 hr	Teratogenicity seen in animals and humans; no specific pattern observed. May cause fetal harm	Stop 2–3 months prior to conception (can consider shorter washout period for siponimod and ponesimod); consider switch to alternate DMT prior to conception to avoid rebound disease or bridge with IV steroids
Dimethyl fumarate/diroximel fumarate/ monomethyl fumarate	1 hr	Increased spontaneous abortion in animals; not reported in humans	Stop at positive pregnancy test
Teriflunomide	18–19 days	Teratogenicity seen in animals; precursor leflunomide is a known human teratogen; no malformations in humans observed thus far	Stop at least 2 years prior to conception, or utilize accelerated elimination protocol with cholestyramine

TABLE 7.1 **Continued**

Disease-Modifying Agent	Drug Half-Life	Fetal and Maternal Risks	Pregnancy Recommendations
Cladribine	24 hr	Teratogenicity seen in animals, based on mechanism of action, concern for fetal harm during pregnancy	Wait at least 6 months prior to conception
Natalizumab	7–15 days	Reduce neonatal survival at supratherapeutc doses in primates; transient hematologic abnormalities in late pregnancy exposure in humans	Switch to B-cell-depleting agent prior to conception, or in select cases can dose during pregnancy every 6–8 weeks with last dose ~30–34 weeks of gestation
Alemtuzumab	12 days	Increased rates of fetal loss, decreased B and T lymphocytes in offspring in animals; no human malformations seen, but thyroid monitoring necessary for mother throughout pregnancy; no evidence for spontaneous abortion or birth defects	Wait at least 4 months from last dose prior to conception attempts .
Rituximab/ ocrelizumab/ ublituximab/ ofatumumab	22 days/ 26 days/ 22 days/ 16 days	No human malformations seen; transient B-cell depletion in human neonates and animals following pregnancy exposure No data for ublituximab given recent approval	Wait ~2–3 months after infusion prior to conception attempts; for ofatumumab, time monthly injection to menses and stop when pregnant

DMT, disease-modifying therapy.

doses as high as 40 times the normal dose. This effect has not been seen in humans. There is no animal evidence of teratogenicity, and the large macromolecule is unlikely to be able to cross the placenta in any significant amount.

Glatiramer Acetate (Copaxone)

Glatiramer acetate has been safe in animals, and thus far in more than 500 human pregnancies, there has been no association with low birth weight, congenital anomaly, preterm birth, or spontaneous abortion. Currently, some neurologists treat women with glatiramer acetate during pregnancy. Glatiramer acetate does not cross the placenta.

Dimethyl Fumarate (Tecfidera)/Diroximel Fumarate (Vumerity)/ Monomethyl Fumarate (Bafiertam)

Evidence from animal studies suggests that dimethyl fumarate does cross the placenta. Animals, given the highest dose tested, showed an increased rate of spontaneous abortion as well as lower fetal weight and delayed ossification. Despite these studies, in a case series of 45 women exposed to dimethyl fumarate in early pregnancy, no significant adverse effects were found. Importantly, these medications have a very short half-life (see Table 7.1), ensuring that the drug is rapidly eliminated from the body soon after therapy is discontinued.

TABLE 7.2 **Disease-Modifying Therapy and Breastfeeding**

Disease-Modifying Agent	Lactation Data	DMT Compatibility With Breastfeeding
Interferon-β-1b and -β -1a	Low concentration in breast milk	Yes
Glatiramer acetate	None to low concentration in breast milk	Yes
Fingolimod/siponimod/ ozanimod/ponesimod	No data; concern that it would be detectable due to low molecular weight	No
Dimethyl fumarate/ diroximel fumarate/ monomethyl fumarate	Minimal data; concern that it would be detectable due to low molecular weight	No

TABLE 7.2 **Continued**

Disease-Modifying Agent	Lactation Data	DMT Compatibility With Breastfeeding
Teriflunomide	Detected in studies of animal milk; no human data	No
Cladribine	Low levels based on one case report	No
Natalizumab	Low concentration based on case series	Yes
Alemtuzumab	No data in humans; detected in animal milk; given high molecular weight, suspected low concentration	Yes, with caution
Rituximab/ocrelizumab/ublituximab/ofatumumab	Undetectable or low concentrations (ocrelizumab, rituximab); no data for ofatumumab or ublituximab, but given high molecular weights, low concentrations suspected	Yes

DMT, disease-modifying therapy.

Fingolimod (Gilenya)/Siponimod (Mayzent)/Ozanimod (Zeposia)/Ponesimod (Ponvory)

Fingolimod crosses the placenta and is secreted in breast milk. In animal studies, there is evidence for both teratogenicity and embryolethality. Fetal malformations and complications included ventricular septal defect, persistent truncus arteriosus, and fetal death. In a limited number of human pregnancies, there seems to be a slightly higher rate of spontaneous abortion, as well as malformations such as acrania, a malformation of the tibia, and tetralogy of Fallot. Currently, it is advised that patients stop fingolimod use at least 2 months prior to conceiving. There are no data on siponimod, ozanimod, or ponesimod, but the teratogenicity is believed to be a class effect among the S1P receptor modulators, and these medications should be stopped prior to conception.

Teriflunomide (Aubagio)

In animal studies, teriflunomide had significant teratogenicity, causing fetal abnormalities such as craniofacial, axial, and appendicular skeletal malformations in pregnant rats and rabbits. Despite these findings, of the recorded human pregnancies with exposure to teriflunomide, the rate of spontaneous abortion was not different from that for the general population, and no serious malformations were reported. However, caution is still advised. In addition to its ability to cross the placenta, teriflunomide is also present in the semen of men taking the drug. Teriflunomide may stay present in the body for as long as 24 months, but it can be eliminated with a washout protocol using cholestyramine to eliminate the drug.

Cladribine (Mavenclad)

Given that this medication inhibits DNA synthesis, it is contraindicated during pregnancy, and there are limited data on pregnancy outcomes. A small study evaluated 39 pregnancies: 17 had exposure to cladribine 6 months prior to last menstrual period (LMP), and 22 had exposure 6 months after their LMP. There were overall similar pregnancy outcomes between the groups, although there was one congenital abnormality in the group that received cladribine within 6 months of LMP.

Natalizumab (Tysabri)

According to the Tysabri Pregnancy Exposure Registry, which reported 375 pregnancies resulting in 314 live births, the rates of miscarriage and malformation were not increased compared to those for the general population. However, in animal studies, supratherapeutic doses of natalizumab have been shown to decrease fertility and reduce neonatal survival. Natalizumab crosses the placenta in the second trimester and is secreted at low levels in breast milk. However, it is unclear whether this monoclonal antibody is absorbed through the infant's gastrointestinal mucosa. Given the possibility for severe rebound of MS disease activity with natalizumab discontinuation, if a patient conceives while on natalizumab, it is reasonable to consider its continuation during pregnancy. If continued during pregnancy, it is still unclear when it should be stopped to mitigate risk of neonatal hematologic abnormalities, but most experts recommend dosing every 6–8 weeks during pregnancy and then stopping at approximately 30–34 weeks of gestation.[7]

Rituximab (Rituxan)/Ocrelizumab (Ocrevus)/Ublituximab (Briumvi)/Ofatumumab (Kesimpta)

Rituximab does cross the placenta according to evidence from animal studies; however, these studies showed no evidence of increased risk of miscarriage or teratogenicity. Similarly, studies in humans on ocrelizumab and ofatumumab showed no negative pregnancy outcomes. One class effect that has been seen in both animal studies and humans is transient newborn B-cell depletion. The risk of B-cell depletion in the newborn appears to be higher when the mother is exposed to the drug during the second or third trimester. Therefore, B-cell-depleting medications are not typically continued during pregnancy for women with MS. There are no data yet on ublituximab given its recent approval; however, it likely has similar characteristics to the other B-cell-depleting monoclonal antibodies.

Alemtuzumab (Lemtrada)

This medication is only used in patients with very aggressive or refractory MS. In animal studies, early administration of alemtuzumab resulted in increased rates of fetal loss, as well as decreased B and T lymphocytes at birth. It is advised that women should avoid conception for at least 4 months after the infusion. In a case series of 104 human patients treated with alemtuzumab and 139 pregnancies, no increased rates of miscarriage or malformations were observed. Almost all of these pregnancies (except 6) were conceived at least 4 months after the alemtuzumab infusion. There was one case of neonatal thyrotoxic crisis that resolved with appropriate treatment.

Breastfeeding

Several studies have suggested that breastfeeding may influence postpartum relapse rate, but the true effect continues to be debated. A small study of women with MS suggested that exclusive breastfeeding might protect against postpartum relapse, possibly through promoting ongoing anti-inflammatory changes. However, a similar study with a much larger pregnancy cohort failed to produce the same findings. In addition, in the PRIMS study, breastfeeding was ultimately considered to have no effect on postpartum relapses or disability. Some suggest that although women who breastfeed appear to do better, these fata may preselect for women with milder disease. Further research is needed to assess whether breastfeeding may alter postpartum magnetic resonance imaging disease activity.

Although there are still many questions, the available evidence suggests that breastfeeding is safe and possibly even beneficial for MS patients. Therefore, although each case should be considered individually, the choice to breastfeed should be generally supported. Specific information about each DMT and breastfeeding is given in Table 26.2. Drugs with higher molecular weight are overall less likely to pass into breast milk. Monoclonal antibodies are large molecules, and if they do pass into breast milk, they are likely be degraded in the infant's gastro-intestinal track.

Assisted Reproductive Technology in Multiple Sclerosis

In general, MS patients are not thought to have decreased fertility as a result of the disease. However, many MS patients are turning to assisted reproductive technology (ART) for various reasons, including delays in childbearing due to their disease and sexual dysfunction.[8]

Although a few small early studies have suggested that there may be an increased risk of relapse with gonadotropin-releasing hormone agonists and recombinant follicle-stimulating hormone,[4] larger published studies did not show an elevated risk of relapse with ART. Women with MS should be counseled that if they need ART, there are no contraindications from their MS.[5]

Counseling Women on Multiple Sclerosis Risk in Their Children

Like many other diseases, MS is thought to occur due to some combination of genes and environmental risk factors. Children of women with MS have a 3–5% lifetime risk of developing the disease. Although this is a greater risk than that for those with no family history, it also means that there is a 95–97% chance a child will not be affected. Clinicians can provide patients with the facts and statistics, but there is still a lot to be learned, and this is currently an active area of research.

KEY POINTS TO REMEMBER

- The rate of relapse in MS decreases during pregnancy, especially during the third trimester, but there is a significant increase in relapse rate in the first 3 months postpartum.
- Disease-modifying therapies are generally discontinued during pregnancy.
- The use of B-cell-depleting monoclonal antibodies prior to pregnancy is associated with lower postpartum relapse rate.
- Breastfeeding is generally recommended, although many DMTs should be avoided while breastfeeding.

References

1. Confavreux C, Hutchinson M, Hours MM, et al. Rate of pregnancy-related relapse in multiple sclerosis. Pregnancy in Multiple Sclerosis Group. *N Engl J Med*. 1998;339(5):285–2291.
2. Vukusic S, Hutchinson M, Hours M, et al. Pregnancy and multiple sclerosis (the PRIMS study): Clinical predictors of post-partum relapse. *Brain*. 2004;127(Pt 6):1353–1360.
3. Hellwig K, Haghikia A, Rockhoff M, Gold R. Multiple sclerosis and pregnancy: Experience from a nationwide database in Germany. *Ther Adv Neurol Disord*. 2012;5(5):247–253.
4. Correale J, Farez MF, Ysrraelit MC. Increase in multiple sclerosis activity after assisted reproduction technology. *Ann Neurol*. 2012;72(5):682–694.
5. Graham EL, Bakkensen JB, Anderson A, et al. Inflammatory activity after diverse fertility treatments: A multicenter analysis in the modern multiple sclerosis treatment era. *Neurol Neuroimmunol Neuroinflamm*. 2023;10(3):e200106.

6. Hellwig K, Tokic M, Thiel S, et al. Multiple sclerosis disease activity and disability following discontinuation of natalizumab for pregnancy. *JAMA Netw Open* 2022;5:e2144750.

7. Razaz N, Piehl F, Frisell T, Langer-Gould AM, McKay KA, Fink K. Disease activity in pregnancy and postpartum in women with MS who suspended rituximab and natalizumab. *Neurol Neuroimmunol Neuroinflamm.* 2020;7:e903.

8. Krysko KM, Dobson R, Alroughani R, et al. Family planning considerations in people with multiple sclerosis. *Lancet Neurol.* 2023;22(4):350–366.

8 A Mother Who Could Not See Her Baby

Sarah Conway and Tamara B. Kaplan

A 30-year-old woman, at 28 weeks gestation, was brought to the emergency department (ED) because she was "not feeling well" and was diagnosed with severe preeclampsia. She subsequently had a caesarian section. Three weeks postpartum, she had intractable hiccups, as well as nausea and vomiting. Two weeks later, she woke up with decreased vision in her right eye ("80% dark") and pain with eye movements. Ophthalmology evaluation revealed that her visual acuity (VA) was finger-counting right eye (OD) and 20/15 left eye (OS). Magnetic resonance imaging of the brain revealed right optic neuritis (ON). She was treated with intravenous (IV) steroids but had no clinical improvement. Plasmapheresis was initiated, and by the third session, she obtained significant improvement. Her laboratory workup was notable for anti-aquaporin-4 (AQP4) antibodies.

What do you do now?

NEUROMYELITIS OPTICA SPECTRUM DISORDERS IN PREGNANCY

AQP4 Antibodies Are the Hallmark of Neuromyelitis Optica Spectrum Disorders

Neuromyelitis optica spectrum disorders (NMOSD) belong to a group of relapsing neurological syndromes characterized by significant morbidity and mortality. The disease happens due to central nervous system (CNS) inflammation and necrosis, which is, in most cases, mediated by antibodies targeting AQP4.

AQP4 is a water channel present in many tissues (CNS, kidneys, muscle, and others) but most greatly expressed on the foot processes of astrocytes. Compared to other organs, the CNS has a much larger content of AQP4, especially in optic nerves, the spinal cord, and certain areas of the brainstem. Along with differences in complement cascade regulation in the CNS compared to other tissues, the greater expression of AQP4 is probably responsible for the disease's common manifestations of ON, transverse myelitis, and area postrema syndrome (intractable nausea/vomiting and/or hiccups). Other brainstem syndromes, narcolepsy, and symptomatic cerebral lesions are also possible but much less common.

Clinical Clues in NMOSD

NMOSD shows a marked female preponderance (6F:1M) and may affect patients of childbearing age. Compared to multiple sclerosis (MS), NMOSD is also more common in non-White populations. As exemplified by the case of the 30-year-old patient, the consideration of a potential diagnosis of NMOSD begins with an indicative clinical syndrome; in this case, her intractable hiccups as well as nausea and vomiting raise the concern for the area postrema syndrome, which is part of the diagnostic criteria for NMOSD. NMOSD usually leads to a more severe ON (VA less than 20/200) with poor recovery, and the optic nerve lesions are more likely to be extensive and with chiasmatic involvement compared to ON in MS.

Patients who are seropositive for anti-AQP4 antibodies (also known as NMO-IgG) are very likely to have NMOSD relapses. The typical myelitis in NMOSD is complete (motor, sensory, and loss of sphincter control) and longitudinally extensive (more than three spinal cord segments). In contrast, MS patients most often have partial spinal cord syndromes, often with sensory abnormalities only. MS-related spinal cord lesions are usually small and peripherally located. Pain and paroxysmal tonic spasms are also more frequent in NMOSD.

The area postrema syndrome happens in almost half of NMO patients along the disease course, often as the initial presentation. "Intractable" nausea, vomiting, and hiccups may occur in isolation or herald the onset of other syndromes, as was the case with our patient.

Planning Pregnancy (I): NMOSD Increases Risk of Miscarriages and Preeclampsia

When counseling a patient with NMOSD who wants to get pregnant, the risk of complications must be discussed. In a study of 40 AQP4-seropositive women with 85 informative pregnancies, there were 11 pregnancies (13%) that ended in miscarriages.[1] Of those, 7 were in the first trimester, 1 in the second trimester, and 3 at an unknown time within the first 24 weeks. Six of 14 pregnancies (43%) after NMOSD clinical onset ended in miscarriages, compared to 5 of 71 pregnancies (7%) that happened before NMOSD onset. In the studied cohort, there was no association between antiphospholipid antibodies and miscarriage rates. It is likely that patients with more "active" disease will have more complications. The mean annualized relapse ratio from the 9 months preconception to the end of pregnancy was higher in the miscarriage subgroup than in the viable pregnancy subgroup (0.707 vs. 0.100, $p = .01$).

Pertinent to the case described, in the same NMOSD pregnancy study, 113 informative pregnancies in 57 women were included in the analysis of the influence of NMOSD on the risk of preeclampsia. The authors found that 13 cases of preeclampsia were distributed among 11 women, corresponding to a preeclampsia rate of 11%. The incidence of preeclampsia in pregnancies occurring before and after NMOSD was similar. Miscarriage in the most recent pregnancy and the presence of multiple other autoimmune diseases were associated with an increased risk of preeclampsia, and no significant association was found between preeclampsia risk and maternal age.

Placenta expresses AQP4, and autoimmunity may be responsible for the pathogenesis of preeclampsia and/or miscarriages. Placental AQP4 expression is high during mid-gestation and progressively decreases with advancing pregnancy. In animal studies, injected anti-AQP4 antibodies bind to mouse placental AQP4, activate proteins of the complement system, and cause inflammatory cell infiltration into the placenta, leading to tissue necrosis.

In addition, more than 20% of patients with NMOSD have coexisting autoimmune disease such as systemic lupus erythematosus, antiphospholipid syndrome, and myasthenia gravis, which also can impact both mother and fetus.[2]

Planning Pregnancy (II): Increased Risk of NMOSD Relapses Postpartum

In addition to having an increased risk for pregnancy complications, patients with NMOSD also have risk of relapse in the first 3 months of the postpartum period, compared to 0–9 months preconception. Withdrawal of pregnancy-related immunological tolerance mechanisms mediated by regulatory T cells may induce an immunological and clinical rebound effect and explain such increase of relapses.[3]

NMOSD Management During Pregnancy and Postpartum

Based on case series and expert opinion, treating NMOSD attacks with steroids and plasmapheresis during pregnancy or postpartum is appropriate, and the incidence of side effects or complications of such therapies does not seem to be affected by pregnancy. It is generally recommended to treat an NMOSD attack with 5 days of 1 g of IV methylprednisolone, and if no significant and immediate response is seen, patients should be started on plasmapheresis sessions every other day for a total of five to seven exchanges.

Immunosuppressive agents are the mainstream method of preventing attacks related to NMOSD. In 2019, three medications to prevent NMOSD attacks were approved by the U.S. Food and Drug Administration: satralizumab, a humanized monoclonal to the interleukin-6 receptor; inebilizumab, a humanized monoclonal antibody to CD19 B cells; and eculizumab, a humanized monoclonal antibody to C5 of the complement cascade. Satralizumab is approved for both seropositive and seronegative NNMOSD, whereas inebilizumab and eculizumab are approved for only seropositive NMOSD.[4] Other medications, including azathioprine, mycophenolate mofetil, and rituximab, are often used.[5] Limited data from literature and from registries of other antibody-mediated diseases show that azathioprine, eculizumab, anti-B-cell therapy (rituximab and inebilizumab), and steroids are the preferred agents to use during pregnancy after risk–benefit discussion. Data on the use of eculizumab and rituximab during pregnancy are drawn from studies of eculizumab in paroxysmal nocturnal hemoglobinuria and rituximab in myasthenia gravis, with no new safety concerns reported. Because inebilizumab is a newer medication, there are no specific data on pregnancy, but based on use of other anti-B-cell monoclonal antibodies, it can be continued during pregnancy if needed.[6]

If a patient is in good control of her disease (no relapses for at least a year) and decides to become pregnant, she should undergo monitoring for preeclampsia and NMOSD relapses. In general, due to the severity of NMOSD attacks, we recommend continuing immunosuppression during pregnancy. If immunosuppression was not continued during pregnancy, it should be resumed as soon as delivery occurs.

There are no studies on lactation and NMOSD. The concentration of any immunoglobulin G in breast milk is very low and generally not absorbed through the intestinal mucosa of the baby. Regarding other common medications used in NMOSD, steroids and azathioprine are detected in breast milk, rarely causing transient neutropenia to the baby.

KEY POINTS TO REMEMBER

- NMOSD is a severe neurological disease, and pathogenic anti-AQP4 antibodies are present in most patients.
- NMOSD increases the risk of miscarriages and preeclampsia.
- Patients with NMOSD have a higher risk of relapses in the first 3 months postpartum.
- Immunosuppression is the mainstream method of treatment of NMOSD and should be continued during pregnancy due to severity of NMOSD relapses.

References

1. Nour M, Nakashima I, Coutinho E, et al. Pregnancy outcomes in aquaporin-4–positive neuromyelitis optica spectrum disorder. *Neurology*. 2016;86(1):79–87.
2. Götestam Skorpen C, Hoeltzenbein M, Tincani A, et al. The EULAR points to consider for use of antirheumatic drugs before pregnancy, and during

pregnancy and lactation. *Ann Rheum Dis.* 2016;75:795–810. doi:10.1136/annrheumdis-2015-208840

3. Leite MI, Panahloo Z, Harrison N, Palace J. A systematic literature review to examine the considerations around pregnancy in women of child-bearing age with myelin oligodendrocyte glycoprotein antibody-associated disease (MOGAD) or aquaporin 4 neuromyelitis optica spectrum disorder (AQP4+ NMOSD). *Mult Scler Relat Disord.* 2023;75:104760. doi:10.1016/j.msard.2023.104760

4. Mao-Draayer Y, Thiel S, Mills EA, et al. Neuromyelitis optica spectrum disorders and pregnancy: Therapeutic considerations. *Nat Rev Neurol.* 2020;16:154–170.

5. Vodopivec I, Matiello M, Prasad S. Treatment of neuromyelitis optica. *Curr Opin Ophthalmol.* 2015;26(6):476–483.

6. Vishnevetsky A, Kaplan TB, Levy M. Transitioning immunotherapy in neuromyelitis optica spectrum disorder–when and how to switch. *Expert Opin Biol Ther.* 2022;22(11):1393–1404.

9 Myelin Oligodendrocyte Glycoprotein Antibody-Associated Disease

Sarah Conway and Tamara B. Kaplan

A 32-year-old female presents to the emergency room with numbness in both of her feet that over the course of a week ascends upwards to below her umbilicus. She also develops urinary retention. She was evaluated in the emergency room and found to have a T10 sensory level and hyperreflexia. She had an MRI of the cervical and thoracic spine that showed a longitudinally extensive enhancing T2 lesion from T9 to T12 involving the conus. She had a lumbar puncture that showed 50 white blood cells/mm^3 with a lymphocytic predominance and a total protein of 40 mg/dl. Oligoclonal bands were negative. She was treated with 5 days of intravenous methylprednisolone for longitudinally extensive transverse myelitis. On day 5 of her hospitalization, her serum myelin oligodendrocyte glycoprotein test came back positive at a titer of 1:1,000. Prior to this hospital admission, she and her partner were planning pregnancy.

What do you do now?

CLINICAL FEATURES AND EPIDEMIOLOGY OF MYELIN OLIGODENDROCYTE GLYCOPROTEIN ANTIBODY-ASSOCIATED DISEASE

Myelin oligodendrocyte glycoprotein antibody-associated disease (MOGAD) is an inflammatory disorder of the central nervous system characterized by transverse myelitis and optic neuritis, and in children a common manifestation is acute disseminated encephalomyelitis (ADEM). MOG is a protein on the surface of oligodendrocytes and is highly immunogenic. Widespread testing for the MOG antibody was not available until 2017. It is likely that many cases of seronegative neuromyelitis optica spectrum disorder (NMOSD) in the past were in retrospect MOGAD.

Approximately 50% of cases of MOGAD are in children. Unlike multiple sclerosis (MS) and NMOSD, there is a relatively equal female-to-male ratio in MOGAD, and some MOG patients, especially children, may have a monophasic course.

Optic neuritis in MOGAD can overlap clinically with optic neuritis seen in MS and NMOSD. Like optic neuritis in NMOSD, MOGAD optic neuritis is typically severe, with most cases having optic disc edema. However, unlike optic neuritis associated with NMOSD, the recovery from MOGAD optic neuritis is typically excellent. Transverse myelitis associated with MOGAD is often accompanied by longitudinally extensive transverse myelitis on magnetic resonance imaging (MRI), which is characteristically located centrally in the spinal cord and preferentially involves the conus and gray matter.

Children with MOGAD commonly present with ADEM, which is characterized by encephalopathy and large, poorly demarcated lesions on MRI. There are also some newer phenotypes of MOGAD, including cerebral cortical encephalitis and seizures. Many cases of MOGAD have significant improvement on MRI over time, which is another distinguishing feature from MS and NMOSD.[1]

Diagnostic criteria for MOGAD were proposed in 2023 and require a core clinical demyelinating event (optic neuritis, myelitis, ADEM, cerebral unifocal or multifocal deficits, brainstem or cerebellar deficits, or cerebral cortical encephalitis often with seizures) in addition to a positive MOG-IgG test by a cell-based assay in the serum. If the serum titer is >1:100, the diagnosis can be made. If the titer is low positive, or negative but positive in the cerebrospinal fluid, then additional supporting clinical or MRI features are required.[2]

Treatment of MOGAD

Acute treatment of MOGAD attacks includes intravenous steroids and/ or intravenous immunoglobulin (IVIG) and plasma exchange. Patients with MOGAD tend to be very steroid responsive, and may relapse with steroid withdrawal, so longer oral corticosteroid tapers over months are recommended after an initial attack.[3]

There are no data from randomized clinical trials on maintenance therapies in MOGAD, although there are ongoing clinical trials. There is also practice variation regarding who should be put on preventative immunosuppression, although persistent seropositivity for MOG antibody is likely a risk factor for relapsing disease. For prevention of an attack in MOGAD, maintenance IVIG has the most impact on relapse reduction.[4] Mycophenolate mofetil and azathioprine have also been used. B-cell-depleting therapies such as rituximab have been used in MOGAD but tend to be less efficacious compared to their use in aquaporin-4-positive NMOSD.

Pregnancy Considerations in MOGAD

Given MOGAD is rare and a more recently recognized distinct clinical condition, data on pregnancy are limited. No studies have examined MOGAD and fertility; however, unlike NMOSD, MOGAD is not associated with other autoimmune diseases and medical comorbidities that can negatively impact fertility and pregnancy outcomes, so we suspect there would be no influence on fertility. There are minimal data on pregnancy outcomes in MOGAD. One study on 21 MOGAD pregnancies found that 18 had term deliveries (1 premature delivery and 2 elective abortions were reported). No spontaneous abortion or congenital malformations were described.[5]

There is inconclusive data in terms of MOGAD relapse rates during pregnancy and postpartum. One study that included 30 MOGAD pregnancies reported a similar relapse rate during pregnancy compared to prepregnancy.[6] Another study on 25 pregnancies in patients with MOGAD from a multicenter French cohort found a lower rate of relapse during pregnancy.[7] Two studies found an increase in relapse rate postpartum similar to what is seen in MS and NMOSD,[5,6] and one study found a lower relapse rate postpartum.[7] Additional larger prospective studies are needed on MOGAD during pregnancy and the postpartum period.

The safety of immunosuppressants for MOGAD during pregnancy can be extrapolated from other disease conditions. In general, rituximab, azathioprine, and IVIG are treatments of choice during pregnancy, whereas mycophenolate mofetil has high rates of teratogenicity and should be avoided.[8]

> **KEY POINTS TO REMEMBER**
>
> - MOGAD is an inflammatory disorder of the central nervous system characterized by transverse myelitis and optic neuritis, and in children a common manifestation is ADEM.
> - MOGAD attacks respond very well to steroids and/or IVIG.
> - There are limited and mixed data on MOGAD in pregnancy. There may be a higher risk of relapse postpartum.

References

1. Cacciaguerra L, Redenbaugh V, Chen JJ, et al. Timing and predictors of T2-lesion resolution in patients with myelin oligodendrocyte glycoprotein antibody-associated disease. *Neurology.* 2023;101(13):e1376–e1381.

2. Banwell B, Bennett JL, Marignier R, et al. Diagnosis of myelin oligodendrocyte glycoprotein antibody-associated disease: International MOGAD Panel proposed criteria. *Lancet Neurol.* 2023;22(3):268–282.

3. Chwalisz BK, Levy M. The treatment of myelin oligodendrocyte glycoprotein antibody disease: A state-of-the-art review. *J Neuroophthalmol.* 2022;42(3):292–296.

4. Chen JJ, Flanagan EP, Bhatti MT, et al. Steroid-sparing maintenance immunotherapy for MOG-IgG associated disorder. *Neurology.* 2020;95(2):e111–e120.

5. Wang L, Zhou L, ZhangBao J, et al. Neuromyelitis optica spectrum disorder: Pregnancy-related attack and predictive risk factors. *J Neurol Neurosurg Psychiatry.* 2020;92(1):53–61.

6. Collongues N, Alves Do Rego C, Bourre B, et al. Pregnancy in patients with AQP4-Ab, MOG-Ab, or double-negative neuromyelitis optica disorder. *Neurology.* 2021;96(15):e2006–e2015.

7. Carra-Dallière C, Rollot F, Deschamps R, et al. Pregnancy and post-partum in patients with myelin-oligodendrocyte glycoprotein antibody-associated disease. *Mult Scler*. 2023;29(2):270–276.

8. Coscia LA, Armenti DP, King RW, Sifontis NM, Constantinescu S, Moritz MJ. Update on the teratogenicity of maternal mycophenolate mofetil. *J Pediatr Genet*. 2015;4(2):42–55.

10 Autoimmune Encephalitis

Sarah Conway and Tamara B. Kaplan

A 21-year-old female is brought to the emergency room by her mother after experiencing new-onset auditory and visual hallucinations. She was evaluated, and after basic labs and a toxicology screen, she was started on haloperidol and discharged with outpatient psychiatric follow-up. One week later, she had a witnessed generalized tonic–clonic seizure and went back to the hospital. At that time, her bizarre behaviors and hallucinations worsened despite the haloperidol. She also was febrile. She had a lumbar puncture, which had 30 white blood cells/mm^3 with a lymphocytic predominance and a total protein of 41 mg/dl. MRI brain was normal. Electroencephalogram (EEG) showed delta brush pattern. She was treated with levetiracetam and also empirically with intravenous acyclovir until herpes simplex virus (HSV) testing from the cerebrospinal fluid (CSF) came back negative. Later in her hospitalization, CSF anti-*N*-methyl-d-aspartate (anti-NMDA) antibodies came back positive.

What do you do now?

Anti-NMDA receptor encephalitis is an immune-mediated disorder characterized by prominent psychiatric manifestations, including anxiety, psychosis, and catatonia, as well as sleep disorders, memory deficits, seizures, dyskinesias, and autonomic and language dysfunction. Although anti-NMDA receptor encephalitis is rare, it is the most prevalent autoimmune encephalitis. Females are more likely to be affected than males.[1] The most common age range is 25–35 years. Diagnosis is based on clinical findings as well as the presence of anti-NMDA antibodies in the serum or CSF. Testing for the anti-NMDA antibody is more sensitive in the CSF than in the serum. Patients who present with the above symptoms and for whom there is concern for autoimmune encephalitis should be evaluated with CSF testing, as well as brain MRI and EEG. CSF testing in anti-NMDA receptor encephalitis typically shows a lymphocytic pleocytosis, although if done early on CSF studies it can be normal. Most EEGs in patients with anti-NMDA receptor encephalitis are abnormal. The most common patterns are generalized rhythmic delta activity as well as extreme delta brush.[2] MRI brain can be normal or can show T2 hyperintense lesions most commonly in the hippocampus.

Some cases of anti-NMDA encephalitis can be triggered by preceding HSV encephalitis. This is believed to be due to the virus' involvement of limbic structures that have high concentrations of NMDA receptors. Other cases can be triggered by malignancies, most commonly ovarian teratomas. In a patient who tests positive for anti-NMDA, it is imperative to screen for malignancy, including whole-body computed tomography, as well as transvaginal ultrasonography for women and testicular ultrasound for men.

Specific diagnostic criteria for probable anti-NMDA receptor encephalitis were proposed in 2016[3] and can be made when all three of the following are met:

1. Rapid onset (less than 3 months) of at least four of the six major groups of symptoms: abnormal psychiatric or cognitive dysfunction, speech dysfunction, seizures, movement disorders, decreased level of consciousness, and autonomic dysfunction or central hypoventilation

2. At least one of the following study results: abnormal EEG, or CSF with pleocytosis or oligoclonal bands
3. Reasonable exclusion of other disorders

TREATMENT

In anti-NMDA encephalitis, the antibody itself is believed to be pathogenic. First-line therapies include high-dose steroids, and if no response or in particularly severe cases, either intravenous immunoglobulin (IVIG) or plasmapheresis is recommended. Second-line therapies include rituximab. If a teratoma is found, it should be removed. Patients with delayed diagnosis and those without a tumor tend to have worse outcomes.[4]

ANTI-NMDA ENCEPHALITIS AND PREGNANCY

Due to the rarity of anti-NMDA encephalitis, information on pregnancy outcomes comes from case series. The largest case series to date was published in 2020 and included outcomes on 11 patients and a literature review of 21 additional cases.[5] Of the 11 patients in the case series, 6 patients were diagnosed during pregnancy, and 5 patients became pregnant after diagnosis. There were no obstetrical complications. Ten out of the 11 newborns were healthy, although 6 (55%) were premature. In the literature review of 21 cases, 33% had obstetrical complications (2 died of septic shock, 2 had miscarriages, and in 2 the pregnancies were terminated); 56% of babies were premature, and 81% were born healthy. In this case series and review, immunosuppressive therapy with steroids, IVIG, and plasmapheresis was used during pregnancy in most patients and was well tolerated. Four patients were treated with rituximab during pregnancy without complications. One of these patients also received IV cyclophosphamide 6 weeks prior to delivery. None of the babies had leukopenia or hypogammaglobulinemia. Follow-up data were reported for 8 children at a median of 12 months: 7 (88%) had normal development, and 1 (12%) had cortical dysplasia. This suggests that despite in utero exposure to NMDA, most babies were healthy at birth; however, obstetric complications are common due to the severity of the disease and medical comorbidities.[5] More studies are needed to understand if serum antibody titers in the mother and newborn are associated with developmental abnormalities or neurologic deficits.

> **KEY POINTS TO REMEMBER**
>
> - Anti-NMDA encephalitis typically presents with behavioral/psychiatric change with abnormalities on EEG or on CSF testing.
> - Anti-NMDA encephalitis is associated with malignancy, most commonly ovarian teratoma.
> - Patients who test positive for anti-NMDA should have thorough malignancy screening, including transvaginal ultrasound for women and testicular ultrasound for men.

References

1. Gable MS, Sheriff H, Dalmau J, Tilley DH, Glaser CA. The frequency of autoimmune *N*-methyl-d-aspartate receptor encephalitis surpasses that of individual viral etiologies in young individuals enrolled in the California Encephalitis Project. *Clin Infect Dis.* 2012;54(7):899–904.
2. Jeannin-Mayer S, André-Obadia N, et al. EEG analysis in anti-NMDA receptor encephalitis: Description of typical patterns. *Clin Neurophysiol.* 2019;130(2):289–296.
3. Graus F, Titulaer MJ, Balu R, et al. A clinical approach to diagnosis of autoimmune encephalitis. *Lancet Neurol.* 2016;15(4):391–404.
4. Florance NR, Davis RL, Lam C, et al. Anti-*N*-methyl-d-aspartate receptor (NMDAR) encephalitis in children and adolescents. *Ann Neurol.* 2009;66(1):11–18.
5. Joubert B, García-Serra A, Planagumà J, et al. Pregnancy outcomes in anti-NMDA receptor encephalitis: Case series. *Neurol Neuroimmunol Neuroinflamm.* 2020;7(3):e668.

11 Paraneoplastic Cerebellar Degeneration

Sarah Conway and Tamara B. Kaplan

A 52-year-old female with no past medical history presents with nausea and vomiting that are followed by imbalance and dizziness. She initially attributed her symptoms to a gastrointestinal illness and dehydration, but a few weeks later she had not improved, and she developed double vision and difficulty with hand coordination. She was concerned about these symptoms, so she presented to her primary care physician, who noted nystagmus, appendicular dysmetria, and a wide-based gait. She was later evaluated by a neurologist and had a brain, which was normal. She had a lumbar puncture, which showed five WBCs/mm^3, a total protein of 20 mg/dl, and a normal opening pressure. Cerebrospinal fluid (CSF) flow cytometry and cytology were negative. She had serum and CSF paraneoplastic panels, which ultimately came back positive for anti-Yo (also called Purkinje cell antibody type 1).

What do you do now?

This patient's clinical syndrome is consistent with paraneoplastic cerebellar degeneration (PCD). There are more than 30 different antibodies associated with PCD. The most common associated antibody is anti-Yo, which occurs in approximately 50% of cases.[1] Anti-Yo PCD primarily occurs in patients with breast or other gynecologic cancers and therefore is predominantly a disorder that affects women.

Most cases of PCD predate cancer diagnosis, and occasionally cancers are identified years later. PCD with anti-Yo antibodies presents with a subacute cerebellar syndrome often with appendicular and truncal ataxia, which progresses to nystagmus and oscillopsia, dysarthria, and dysphagia. The symptoms are quite severe, with many patients becoming unable to ambulate independently. Magnetic resonance imaging early in the course can be normal. As the disease progresses, cerebellar atrophy is seen. CSF abnormalities are noted in most patients with paraneoplastic disorders. A study of 53 patients with anti-Yo syndrome found that 51 had abnormal CSF, most with mild pleocytosis, protein elevation, or oligoclonal bands.[2] High levels of white blood cells in the CSF should raise concern for either infection or leptomeningeal disease. If PCD is suspected, a paraneoplastic antibody panel must be done ideally in both serum and CSF. If an antibody is detected, then patients must have a workup for underlying malignancy to include computed tomography scans of the chest, abdomen, and pelvis and, if negative, then also a positron emission tomography scan. In women, it is also important to consider transvaginal ultrasounds and mammograms. If no cancer is found, patients should be rescreened every 6 months. A large study from the Mayo Clinic on patients who tested positive for anti-Yo found that after a median follow-up of 18 months, 88% had cancer detected, the most common type being ovarian cancer (53%), followed by breast cancer (22%), fallopian tube cancer (11%), primary peritoneal cancer (5%), metastases of unknown primary (4%), and other cancer (4%).[3]

MANAGEMENT AND PROGNOSIS OF
ANTI-YO–ASSOCIATED PCD

In anti-Yo–associated PCD, the antibody is intracellular, implicating a cytotoxic T cell response. Treatment focuses on the underlying malignancy and the cytotoxic T cell response. There are no randomized clinical trials to guide therapy. Typically, empiric cyclophosphamide is used with or without steroids or intravenous immunoglobulin. Unfortunately, prognosis is poor, with significant disability. One series found that only 15% of patients had neurologic stabilization or improvement with treatment. That same series found that median survival from onset of neurologic symptoms was 24 months, and only 9% survived for 5 or more years.[3] Other studies report even lower median survival rates of 13 months,[4] and outcomes are likely worse with older age, breast cancer as opposed to ovarian malignancies,[5] and later immunosuppression.

KEY POINTS TO REMEMBER

- PCD is a disabling neurologic disease, often with associated autoantibodies.
- Anti-Yo is the most common autoantibody identified, and its discovery should lead to a workup for occult malignancy with a focus on breast and gynecologic cancers.
- Prognosis is poor, and early treatment with immunosuppression is important to prevent disability.

References

1. O'Brien TJ, Pasaliaris B, D'Apice A, Byrne E. Anti-Yo positive paraneoplastic cerebellar degeneration: A report of three cases and review of the literature. *J Clin Neurosci.* 1995;2(4):316–320.
2. Peterson K, Rosenblum MK, Kotanides H, Posner JB. Paraneoplastic cerebellar degeneration: I. A clinical analysis of 55 anti-Yo antibody-positive patients. *Neurology.* 1992;42(10):1931–1937.
3. McKeon A, Tracy JA, Pittock SJ, Parisi JE, Klein CJ, Lennon VA. Purkinje cell cytoplasmic autoantibody type 1 accompaniments: The cerebellum and beyond. *Arch Neurol.* 2011;68(10):1282–1289.
4. Shams'ili S, Grefkens J, de Leeuw B, et al. Paraneoplastic cerebellar degeneration associated with antineuronal antibodies: Analysis of 50 patients. *Brain.* 2003;126(Pt 6):1409–1418.
5. Rojas I, Graus F, Keime-Guibert F, et al. Long-term clinical outcome of paraneoplastic cerebellar degeneration and anti-Yo antibodies. *Neurology.* 2000;55(5):713–715.

SECTION III

Headache Disorders

12 Hormonal Contraception in a Woman With Headache

Addie Peretz

A 27-year-old woman presents for evaluation of long-standing headaches. She reports headaches began in high school and are usually right hemicranial and throbbing in nature. They are often preceded by shimmering zigzag lines, which occur on of the right side of her vision. These visual phenomena are often followed by right visual field loss. The visual symptoms typically last approximately 20–30 minutes. The headaches are associated with light sensitivity as well as nausea and vomiting. They occur at least once a week and last 24–48 hours. She has previously tried amitriptyline, propranolol, and Excedrin migraine tablets without success. She has not noticed any clear triggers for her headaches. Her past medical history is unremarkable. Her current medications are Ortho Tri-Cyclen and naproxen PRN (i.e., as needed). She drinks alcohol occasionally and smokes cigarettes, about one pack a day. Her examination is normal.

What do you do now?

MIGRAINE AND HORMONAL CONTRACEPTION

This chapter examines key issues around contraception in women with migraine. There is a small increased risk of stroke for women with migraine with aura. The risk is further increased when combined with other risk factors, such as smoking and hypertension. The use of combined oral contraceptive pills (OCPs) contributes independently to stroke risk. This risk appears to be correlated with estrogen in a dose-dependent manner but not with progesterone. Drug–drug interactions between migraine prophylactic medications and OCPs are also critical to consider. The appropriate choice of contraceptive method should be made on an individual basis, taking into account the patient's headache type, medical history, medications, and cerebrovascular risk factors.

Diagnosis

This patient suffers from migraine with aura. Migraine affects 6–18% of the population, with women being affected three times more frequently than men. The prevalence of migraine increases with age such that nearly 29% of women between ages 30 and 39 years experience migraine.[1] Nearly one-third of individuals with migraine experience aura, a transient neurologic phenomena that tends to occur before or during migraine headache. Aura is most commonly visual, although it can involve sensory, motor, and speech disturbances, among other neurologic phenomena. The diagnosis of migraine with aura can be made clinically based on fulfilling criteria delineated in the third edition of the *International Classification of Headache Disorders* (ICHD-3) and shown in Box 12.1. Patients with a new presentation of neurologic disturbance associated with migraine may require neuroimaging with brain magnetic resonance imaging and neck and brain vascular imaging to exclude secondary headaches that can mimic migraine.

Although hormonal contraceptives should not be the mainstay of treatment for migraine, patients may need to take hormonal contraceptives for a variety of reasons, including contraception, endometriosis, menstrual cramping, dysmenorrhea, and menorrhagia. Combined hormonal contraception (CHC) is the most commonly prescribed method of contraception. Of note, the estrogen content of CHCs has decreased over time, with

> **BOX 12.1 Migraine with Aura**
>
> **Description**
>
> Recurrent attacks, lasting minutes, of unilateral fully reversible visual, sensory, or other central nervous system symptoms that usually develop gradually and are usually followed by headache and associated migraine symptoms.
>
> **Diagnostic Criteria**
>
> A. At least two attacks fulfilling criteria B and C
> B. One or more of the following fully reversible aura symptoms:
>   1. Visual
>   2. Sensory
>   3. Speech and/or language
>   4. Motor
>   5. Brainstem
>   6. Retinal
> C. At least three of the following six characteristics:
>   1. At least one aura symptom spreads gradually over ≥5 minutes
>   2. Two or more aura symptoms occur in succession
>   3. Each individual aura symptom lasts 5–60 minutes[1]
>   4. At least one aura symptom is unilateral[2]
>   5. At least one aura symptom is positive[3]
>   6. The aura is accompanied, or followed within 60 minutes, by headache
> D. Not better accounted for by another ICHD-3 diagnosis

current CHCs including 20–25 μg of ethinyl estradiol (EE) compared with first-generation contraceptives that contained as much as 50 μg of EE.

Stroke Risk and Oral Contraceptive Pills

The risk of ischemic stroke (IS) is estimated to be approximately two times higher among patients using estrogen-containing oral contraceptives compared with non-users, in a dose-dependent manner.[2] The absolute risk for IS in women using a CHC is estimated to be low, but it rises dramatically after age 45 years. The risk is exclusively related to estrogen, and there has been no evidence to suggest progesterone alone confers additional risk. A meta-analysis of studies showed 2.75 greater odds of a stroke in a woman with any OCP use.[3] More recent studies examining exclusively low-dose

CHCs have shown a comparable risk. The data for hemorrhagic stroke risk are less consistent. It is known that the risk of stroke with CHC OCPs increases in women who have other traditional stroke risk factors, such as increased age, smoking, and hypertension. For these women, CHCs may not be the best choice of contraception, and aggressive stroke risk factor modification is important.[2]

Stroke Risk in Migraine With Aura and the Role of CHCs

The absolute risk of ischemic stroke for women not using CHC is estimated to be 2.5 strokes per 100,000 women-years in women without migraine, compared with 5.9 strokes per 100,000 women-years in women with migraine with aura and 4 strokes per 100,000 women-years in women with migraine without aura. With CHC use, the risk of stroke increased by 2.5-fold for all groups.[2,4] The absolute risk of IS is small. The Women's Health Study found that there were four additional cases of IS per 10,000 women each year where migraine with aura was the presumed etiology. This study also showed that patients with migraine with aura tend to have transient ischemic attacks and nondisabling strokes. An increased frequency of migraine with aura is associated with an increased risk of stroke.[4] Therefore, the American Heart Association in its guidelines on stroke in women recommends that prophylactic medication should be considered in women who have frequent migraine with aura. In addition, smoking cessation is strongly recommended.[5]

In light of the increased risk of stroke among women on CHCs and the potential additional risk among women with migraine with aura, the World Health Organization and the American Congress of Obstetricians and Gynecologists guidelines consider migraine with aura an absolute contraindication to CHCs.[6] A statement from the International Headache Society in 2000 recommends caution with CHC use in women with migraine, although an individualized approach to CHC use for women with migraine with aura is advised rather than an absolute contraindication.[5] Additional studies are needed to better determine the risk of stroke for women with migraine with aura using current preparations of CHCs because prior studies did not stratify stroke risk by estrogen dose.

Oral Contraceptive Pills' Interactions With Migraine Medications

Practically speaking, medication interaction with OCPs is not significant for most medications used for acute migraine treatment unless these medications are being used in excess. When prescribing a medication for a woman in the childbearing years, the medication safety during pregnancy should be considered. If the medication to be prescribed has potential teratogenic effects, then effective contraception should be discussed. In addition, what effect, if any, the medication may have on their current mode of contraception should also be considered. Table 12.1 shows the common classes of medication used for migraine prophylaxis and those that should be avoided during pregnancy. Table 12.2 shows the effects of common migraine prophylactic medications on OCPs.[7] For the most part, there are no significant interactions except when topiramate is used in doses above 200 mg daily.

TABLE 12.1 **Migraine Preventative Medications and Level of Risk During Pregnancy**

Preferred in pregnancy from a safety perspective: verapamil, cyproheptadine

Second line in pregnancy from a safety perspective: propranolol, amitriptyline

Avoid these medications in pregnancy: topiramate, valproic acid, venlafaxine

TABLE 12.2 **Commonly Used Migraine Preventative Medications and OCP Interaction**

Drug Class	Generic Name	OCP Interaction
Beta blockers	Atenolol, propranolol	No effect
Antiepileptics	Gabapentin	No effect
	Topiramate	Decreases efficacy in doses >200 mg/day
	Valproate	No effect
	Carbamazepine	Reduces estrogen levels
	Oxcarbazepine	Reduces estrogen levels
Calcium channel blocker	Verapamil	No effect
Tricyclic antidepressants	Amitriptyline	No effect

OCP, oral contraceptive pill.

Recommendations to our patient would be the following:

1. She should discontinue the CHC and use either a nonhormonal or a progesterone-only contraceptive method. One highly effective and appropriate contraceptive for this type of patient is the progesterone-only intrauterine device.
2. Given her small but real risk from stroke due to migraine with aura, smoking cessation should be strongly recommended.
3. Prophylactic medication should be offered to her due to the frequency of her migraine attacks. Topiramate would be a reasonable choice. The dose used in migraine prophylaxis, typically targeting 100 mg daily, would not interfere with the efficacy of her contraceptive method. However, a discussion about why an effective contraceptive method is needed is important because topiramate is teratogenic.
4. Acute therapy with a triptan would also be appropriate.
5. She should keep a headache diary to follow her migraine frequency and identify triggers, which would be discussed at her follow-up evaluation.

Migraine and Pregnancy

Discussing our patients' plans for family expansion is critical, especially in light of the teratogenic potential of some of the available migraine treatments. Some medications, such as calcitonin gene-related peptide monoclonal antibody antagonists and onabotulinum toxin A, may need to be stopped months in advance of conception. Many patients also seek preconception counseling to understand how migraine will influence pregnancy outcomes and how pregnancy influences migraine. Approximately 80% of women, particularly women with migraine without aura, will experience an improvement in migraine over the course of pregnancy; typically, pregnant patients experience an improvement beginning around the second or third trimester. This gradual improvement is thought to be related to the steady rise in estrogen over the course of pregnancy.[8] Breastfeeding can also be protective against the recurrence of migraine. With regard to the influence of migraine on pregnancy outcomes, for women with migraine, particularly migraine with aura, there is an increased risk for adverse pregnancy outcomes such as preeclampsia. It is important to monitor closely for signs and symptoms of preeclampsia.

Behavioral and nonpharmacologic strategies should be first-line treatments for treating migraine during pregnancy. Mind–body therapies have evidence for efficacy in treating migraine, and the lack of side effects renders these ideal treatment options to consider. Neuromodulation devices are also a promising migraine treatment during pregnancy because the theoretical risks to mother and fetus are low; however, there are insufficient data to definitively conclude that neuromodulatory devices are safe in pregnancy. Rayhill's article, "Headache in Pregnancy and Lactation," contains a helpful overview of the current knowledge of medication safety and efficacy for treating migraine during pregnancy and is a helpful resource for this information.[8]

KEY POINTS TO REMEMBER

- There is a small risk of stroke related to OCPs that is attributed to estrogen.
- The risk of stroke related to CHCs increases with age and other traditional stroke risk factors. Thus, for women older than age 45 years, especially with other stroke risk factors, another form of contraception should be considered.
- Migraine with aura increases the risk of ischemic stroke by 2.5 times, but the absolute number of strokes is small.
- For women who have migraine with aura, caution is advised with CHCs, with a preference for avoiding or using the lowest dose of estrogen necessary for the patient if there are no other options.
- Migraine, especially migraine without aura, often improves in the second trimester.
- Patients with migraine are at increased risk for preeclampsia.
- When possible, behavioral and nonpharmacologic treatment options such as cognitive–behavioral therapy, biofeedback, and acupuncture should be first-line treatment for women with migraine during pregnancy.

References

1. Buse DC, Loder EW, Gorman JA, et al. Sex differences in the prevalence, symptoms, and associated features of migraine, probable migraine and other severe headache: Results of the American Migraine Prevalence and Prevention (AMPP) study. *Headache*. 2013;53:1278–1299.

2. Sacco S, Merki-Feld GS, Ægidius KL, et al. Hormonal contraceptives and risk of ischemic stroke in women with migraine: A consensus statement from the European Headache Federation (EHF) and the European Society of Contraception and Reproductive Health (ESC). *J Headache Pain*. 2017;18:108.

3. Christensen H, Bushnell C. Stroke in women. *Continuum*. 2020;26:363–385.

4. Tietjen GE, Maly EF. Migraine and ischemic stroke in women: A narrative review. *Headache*. 2020;60:843–863.

5. Bousser MG, Conard J, Kittner S, et al. Recommendations on the risk of ischaemic stroke associated with use of combined oral contraceptives and hormone replacement therapy in women with migraine. The International Headache Society Task Force on Combined Oral Contraceptives & Hormone Replacement Therapy. *Cephalalgia*. 2000;20:155–156.

6. ACOG Committee on Practice Bulletins–Gynecology. ACOG practice bulletin No. 73: Use of hormonal contraception in women with coexisting medical conditions. *Obstet Gynecol*. 2006;107:1453–1472.

7. Hranilovich JA, Kaiser EA, Pace A, Barber M, Ziplow J. Headache in transgender and gender-diverse patients: A narrative review. *Headache*. 2021;61:1040–1050.

8. Rayhill M. Headache in pregnancy and lactation. *Continuum*. 2022;28:72–92.

13 Headache Around Menses

Addie Peretz, Regina Krel, and
Paul G. Mathew

A 26-year-old woman presents with throbbing unilateral headaches with an 8/10 intensity in the visual analog scale. They are associated with photophobia, phonophobia, nausea, and vomiting. She denies visual, sensory, language, or motor disturbances suggesting aura.

Individual attacks last 6–24 hours, and she estimates having seven headache days per month that tend to have a strong menstrual association. The majority of headaches begin 2 days prior to the onset of her menstrual cycle and continue 3 days into menstruation. Her menstrual cycles are regular, occurring approximately every 28-days.

She has no other medical problems and is not taking any medications. She has no allergies, and she denies any tobacco or illicit drug use. There is a family history of migraine involving her mother and maternal grandmother. Her neurological examination was unremarkable.

What do you do now?

MENSTRUALLY RELATED MIGRAINE

Migraine is a disorder with a higher prevalence among women, and is the most disabling condition impacting young women. Nearly 60% of women of reproductive age report an association between migraine and menses, with menses serving as one of the most significant risk factors for migraine without aura.[1,2]

This patient's headaches fulfill criteria for migraine without aura, and *The International Classification of Headache Disorders*, third edition,[1] further characterizes perimenstrual migraine as either pure menstrual migraine (migraine occurring only during menstruation) or menstrually related migraine (perimenstrual migraine attacks and also at other times of the menstrual cycle). In this case, the patient has menstrually related migraine without aura because she experiences some perimenstrual migraine attacks and other attacks outside of her menstrual periods.

MENSTRUALLY RELATED MIGRAINE WITHOUT AURA

The following are diagnostic criteria for menstrually related migraine without aura:

A. Attacks, in a menstruating woman, fulfilling criteria for migraine without aura and criterion B below
B. Occurring on day 1 ± 2 (i.e., days –2 to +3) of menstruation in at least two out of three menstrual cycles, and additionally at other times of the cycle

The prevalence of menstrually related migraine can range from 20% to 60%, whereas pure menstrual migraine occurs in less than 10% of women.[2,3] Menstrual migraine attacks are typically not associated with aura. They tend to be more severe, longer lasting, more refractory to treatment, and are associated with higher rates of functional disability.

A diary or calendar documenting migraine attacks and menstrual cycles should be kept over the course of three consecutive cycles. A diagnosis of menstrually related migraine can be confirmed when two of those menstrual cycles correlate with migraine onset within –2 to +3 days of menses. In contrast to patients of pure menstrual migraine, patients with menstrually related migraine also have attacks at other times during the menstrual cycle.

Studies have demonstrated that the rapid decline in estrogen during the late luteal phase is strongly associated with a migraine attack.[4] Oxytocin and calcitonin gene-related peptide (CGRP) may also play a role in triggering menstrually related migraine attacks.[5]

Treating these more disabling migraine attacks can be challenging. Strategies include (1) employing standard rescue and prophylactic strategies when appropriate, (2) episodic or spot prophylaxis using rescue medications, and (3) hormonal therapy. Triptans and nonsteroidal anti-inflammatory drugs (NSAIDs) have been studied in the setting of menstrually related migraine and can be effective in aborting a migraine attack. Oxytocin agonists, CGRP antagonists, and neuromodulators such as remote electrical neuromodulation (REN) are therapies that may also prove effective treatment options for pure menstrual and menstrually related migraine.[6] Treatment options include the following:

1. Standard acute and prophylactic strategies: Among acute migraine strategies, the following have been studied in the setting of perimenstrual migraine attacks: frovatriptan,[7] naratriptan, zolmitriptan, NSAIDs, ubrogepant, and REN. Prophylactic medications such as CGRP monoclonal antibody therapies and magnesium have also been studied in the setting of menstrual migraine and have demonstrated potential to effectively prevent menstrual migraine, although additional studies are needed to further explore efficacy.[8]

2. Pulse prophylaxis: For patients with predictable menstrual cycles who have few migraine attacks outside of menstruation, pulse prophylaxis can be an effective strategy. NSAIDs such as naproxen and triptans such as frovatriptan have been studied in the setting of pulse prophylaxis for menstrually related migraine. The strategy involves twice daily dosing of either naproxen or frovatriptan 1 or 2 days before the anticipated menstrually related migraine attack, and continuing twice daily dosing for the following 3–5 consecutive days.

3. Hormonal therapy: Hormonal options, such as continuous estrogen with monophasic hormonal contraceptives, can help forestall or disrupt the late luteal phase decline in estrogen and thereby delay or reduce the likelihood of menstrually related migraine attacks. It should be noted that fluctuations in estrogen levels, especially sudden drops, can precipitate migraine. As such, oral contraceptive pills may suppress migraine attacks that would normally occur during menses, but may serve as a trigger during other times of the month in certain patients.[9] Because estrogen-based contraceptives are associated with an increased risk of stroke, and patients who experience migraine with aura carry a slightly increased risk of stroke, physicians should consider the use of progesterone-only formulations.

KEY POINTS TO REMEMBER

- Menstrually related migraine attacks tend to be longer lasting, more debilitating, and more refractory to standard acute treatments than non-menstrual migraine attacks.
- The diagnosis of menstrual migraine is made based on history, physical examination, and analysis of headache diaries/calendars demonstrating a menstrual relationship to migraine attacks in two out of three menstrual cycles. This diagnosis should be made after secondary headaches have been ruled out.
- Pathophysiology of menstrually related migraine is thought to be related to the rate of decline of estrogen in the late luteal phase.
- Perimenstrual prophylaxis with NSAIDs, triptans, or hormones may be beneficial in reducing frequency and intensity of menstrually related migraine attacks.
- Emerging therapies, including CGRP antagonism, oxytocin agonism, and neuromodulation, may be effective in treating menstrually related migraine.

References

1. Headache Classification Committee of the International Headache Society. *The International Classification of Headache Disorders*, 3rd edition. *Cephalalgia*. 2018;38:1–211.

2. MacGregor EA. Migraine management during menstruation and menopause. *Continuum*. 2015;21:990–1003.

3. Pavlović JM. Headache in women. *Continuum*. 2021;27:686–702.

4. Pavlović JM, Allshouse AA, Santoro NF, et al. Sex hormones in women with and without migraine: Evidence of migraine-specific hormone profiles. *Neurology*. 2016;87:49–56.

5. Krause DN, Warfvinge K, Haanes KA, Edvinsson L. Hormonal influences in migraine: Interactions of oestrogen, oxytocin and CGRP. *Nat Rev Neurol*. 2021;17:621–633.

6. Ceriani CEJ, Silberstein SD. Current and emerging pharmacotherapy for menstrual migraine: A narrative review. *Expert Opin Pharmacother*. 2023;24:617–627.

7. Brandes JL, Poole A, Kallela M, et al. Short-term frovatriptan for the prevention of difficult-to-treat menstrual migraine attacks. *Cephalalgia*. 2009;29:1133–1148.

8. Silvestro M, Orologio I, Bonavita S, et al. Effectiveness and safety of CGRP-mAbs in menstrual-related migraine: A real-world experience. *Pain Ther*. 2021;10:1203–1214.

9. Mathew PG, Dun EC, Luo JJ. A cyclic pain: The pathophysiology and treatment of menstrual migraine. *Obstet Gynecol Surv*. 2013 Feb;68(2):130–140.

14 Seeing Spots: Complicated Migraines

Christina R. Catherine

A 37-year-old woman presents to the emergency department with a chief complaint of right hand numbness and tingling that started after she started to see her usual visual aura. Symptoms have been present for almost 2.5 hours now and are associated with a severe, throbbing, unilateral headache, nausea and photophobia. She has a history of migraine with aura but none have ever lasted this long. She took naratriptan without any improvement in symptoms. Past medical history is notable for asthma, anxiety, and irritable bowel syndrome. She reports smoking cigarettes and is taking combined oral contraceptive birth control. Examination is notable for right visual field cut and numbness in the right hand. CT perfusion showed prolonged mean transit time and decreased cerebral blood flow in the left posterior region.

What do you do now?

COMPLICATED OR COMPLEX MIGRAINES

This would be an easy case for the initial physician evaluating her to dismiss her symptoms as a colloquially called "complicated migraine" with possible underlying somatic complaints; however, the persistence of her aura symptoms beyond 60 minutes is a red flag that should prompt further neurological evaluation and imaging. In this case, magnetic resonance imaging of the brain with and without contrast was performed and notable for an acute infarct in the left posterior cerebral artery territory and was consistent with the stroke symptoms that she was experiencing.

The occurrence of a stroke during an attack of migraine with aura is known as migrainous infarction (MI), a rare form of ischemic stroke accounting for 0.5–1.5% of all ischemic strokes and may account for up to 13% of ischemic strokes in younger patients.[1,2] MI has an estimated incidence of 0.8 per 100,000 people and is more common in women. The most commonly affected vascular territory is the posterior circulation (70.6%), with the majority of strokes being small (64.7%).[1] Multiple lesions can be observed in approximately 40% of cases. The formal criteria for MI per *The International Classification of Headache Disorders*, third edition (ICHD-3), is detailed in Box 14.1.

BOX 14.1 **Migrainous Infarction**

Description

One or more migraine aura symptoms occurring in association with an ischemic brain lesion in the appropriate territory demonstrated by neuroimaging, with onset during the course of a typical migraine with aura attack.

Diagnostic Criteria

A. A migraine attack fulfilling criteria B and C
B. Occurring in a patient with migraine with aura and typical of previous attacks except that one or more aura symptoms persists for >60 minutes
C. Neuroimaging demonstrates ischemic infarction in a relevant area
D. Not better accounted for by another ICHD-3 diagnosis

Proposed mechanisms of migraine-associated cerebral infarction include cortical spreading depression, hemodynamic changes/cerebral hypoperfusion, endovascular dysfunction, neurogenic inflammation, arterial vasospasm, transient cerebral edema, and platelet aggregation.[3] Underlying vascular risk factors, the presence of patent foramen ovale, or enhanced atherosclerotic disease have not correlated with an increased risk of stroke in patients with migraine with aura.[4] Cortical spreading depression (CSD) has continued to be the suspected mechanism of migraine aura. CSD occurs as a wave of neuronal depolarization associated with transient (1–2 minutes) cerebral hyperperfusion, followed by neuronal suppression and cerebral hypoperfusion that can last for 1 or 2 hours.[5] This may be accompanied by a 20–30% reduction in cerebral blood flow, which in the right situation may lead to either an ischemic infarct or MI.[5] Vasospasm of large and small vessels has also been documented in several cases of MI.[4]

Independent of MI, migraine with aura has been associated with up to a twofold increased lifetime risk of stroke, whereas patients who only have migraine without aura appear to be comparable to patients without history of migraines (relative risk: 1.56–2.41).[3-5] The reason for this increased risk remains unknown; however, cardiovascular risk factors such as hyperlipidemia, Raynaud phenomenon, hypertension, ischemic heart disease, and myocardial infarction have been found to occur more frequently in patients with migraines than the general population.[3,6] The strongest association between migraine and ischemic stroke is for women younger than age 45 years (relative risk: 2.76–3.65), women who use oral contraceptives (relative risk: 7.02–8.72), and women who smoke (relative risk: 9.03).[5] People who have had a migraine attack within the past 12 months and who have more frequent migraine attacks are also at higher risk of ischemic stroke.[5]

To help mitigate this increased cardiovascular and stroke risk, all patients with migraine should be counseled to abstain or quit smoking. Identified vascular risk factors should be treated appropriately to help mitigate any further increased stroke risk. This includes appropriate follow-up and specialty referral for postpartum women who experienced gestational diabetes, gestational hypertension, or other hypertensive disorders of pregnancy because their risk for future cardiovascular disease is even higher. Women with migraine with aura should also be counseled on the risk of choosing estrogen-containing birth control and recommended to use either nonhormonal options (condoms, copper intrauterine device, or permanent methods) or progesterone-only methods (progesterone-only intrauterine device, mini pill, depot injection, or subdermal implant), depending on their family planning needs.

Interestingly, decreasing migraine attacks with migraine preventative medications does not appear to reduce later cardiovascular or stroke risk.[5] Triptans, nonsteroidal anti-inflammatories, acetaminophen, aspirin, and caffeine are all potential options for acute treatment for migraine with or without aura, depending on the patient's history of stroke and cardiovascular disease. Ergotamines should be avoided in patients with a history of cardiovascular disease or stroke. Opiates and butalbital formulations should be avoided to prevent transformation from episodic to chronic migraine because increased frequency of migraine attacks is associated with increased risk of stroke. Opiates should further be avoided because a large retrospective cohort study that examined older U.S. adults taking opiates versus triptans for acute migraine treatment showed an increased risk of ischemic stroke in the opiate group (adjusted hazard ratio of 1.21 vs. 0.83).[7] The choice of acute treatment options has expanded in recent years, and for migraineurs who have experienced a stroke or other cardiovascular event, calcitonin gene-related peptide inhibitors and serotonin 1F receptor agonists are a potential treatment option without any significant safety issues noted at this time.[5,8]

> **KEY POINTS TO REMEMBER**
>
> - For patients with migraine with aura, there is approximately a twofold increased risk of stroke during their lifetime. This risk is highest for women younger than age 45 years who have migraine with aura, are on estrogen-containing birth control, and who smoke.
> - Migrainous infarction is a rare cause of stroke but should be considered in any patient presenting with an aura that persists for longer than 60 minutes.
> - The etiology for the increased risk of stroke in patients with migraine with aura remains unclear. Several studies have noted

higher rates of vascular risk factors and patent foramen ovale in patients with migraine that may predispose them to higher rates of stroke, although this has not borne out in more recent large-scale studies. Cortical spreading depression, cerebral hypoperfusion, and cerebral vasospasm during migraine with aura may be more significant contributors to higher rates of stroke, especially migrainous infarction.

- Actively managing other cardiovascular risk factors may help lower the risk of stroke in patients who have migraine with aura, such as quitting smoking and treating hypertension and diabetes.

References

1. Vinciguerra L, Cantone M, Lanza G, et al. Migrainous infarction and cerebral vasospasm: Case report and literature review. *J Pain Res*. 2019;12:2941–2950. https://doi.org/10.2147/JPR.S209485

2. Headache Classification Committee of the International Headache Society. *The international classification of headache disorders*. 3rd ed. 2018. https://ichd-3.org/1-migraine/1-4-complications-of-migraine/1-4-3-migrainous-infarction-2

3. Gryglas A, Smigiel R. Migraine and stroke: What's the link? What to do? *Curr Neurol Neurosci Rep*. 2017;17(3):22. doi:10.1007/s11910-017-0729-y

4. Linstra KM, van Os HJA, Ruigrok Y., et al. Sex differences in risk profile, stroke cause, and outcome in ischemic stroke patients with and without migraine. *Front Neurosci*. 2021;15:740639. https://doi.org/10.3389/fnins.2021.740639

5. Øie LR, Kurth T, Gulati S, Dodick D. Migraine and risk of stroke. *J Neurol Neurosurg Psychiatry*. 2020;91:593–604. http://dx.doi.org/10.1136/jnnp-2018-318254

6. Kurth T, Rist PM, Ridker PM, Kotler G, Bubes V, Buring JE. Association of migraine with aura and other risk factors with incident cardiovascular disease in women. *JAMA*. 2020;323(22):2281–2289. doi:10.1001/jama.2020.7172

7. McKinley EC, Lay CL, Rosenson R, et al. Risk for ischemic stroke and coronary heart disease associated with migraine and migraine medication among older adults. *J Headache Pain*. 2021;22:124. https://doi.org/10.1186/s10194-021-01338-z

8. Gomez J, Burish M, Savitz S, McCullough L, Cazaban C. Incidence of ischemic stroke among migraineurs on calcitonin gene-related peptide inhibitors. *Stroke*. 2021;52:AP643. https://doi.org/10.1161/str.52.suppl_1.P643

15 Headaches: When It's Not a Migraine

Arathi Nandyala and Addie Peretz

A 32-year-old woman presents for evaluation of headaches. She describes left retro-orbital pain that is severe and is associated with ipsilateral conjunctival injection, ptosis, and lacrimation. The pain lasts 2 hours per episode, and the headaches have occurred daily for 6–8 weeks. She takes ibuprofen for these headaches without improvement. Her neurologic examination is unremarkable.

What do you do now?

PRIMARY HEADACHE DISORDERS OTHER THAN MIGRAINES

Primary headache disorders, such as tension-type headache and trigeminal autonomic cephalgias (TACs) including cluster headache, occur in both women and men, although the prevalence of these disorders differs in women compared with men (Table 15.1). To date, little is known about the influence of specific hormonal milieus, such as menstruation, hormonal contraceptive use, pregnancy, and menopause, on the severity, frequency, and duration of tension-type headache and TACs. Treatment for tension-type headache and cluster headache is currently the same for women and men, although with further research on the specific gender-influenced manifestations of tension-type headache and cluster headache, gender-informed treatments may emerge.

Trigeminal Autonomic Cephalgias

Cluster Headaches

This patient's headaches meet criteria for cluster headache. There are four types of TACs, whose core features are marked by attacks of side-locked pain in the trigeminal distribution and are associated with ipsilateral cranial autonomic features. Although these are rare compared to tension-type headache and migraine, the severe and disabling nature of these headaches warrants prompt recognition and treatment (Box 15.1). The four types of TACs are distinguished from each other by the duration of each attack and frequency with which the attacks occur. Cluster headache is the most common of the TACs. Unlike in migraine, cluster headache is three times more common in men than women. These severe and disabling headaches are characterized by episodes of sharp, stabbing unilateral head pain lasting 15–180 minutes, with either associated ipsilateral autonomic symptoms or severe agitation.[1] Whereas cluster headache is considered a disease that primarily affects men, women tend to experience the chronic, remitting phenotype more often. To rule out other secondary causes of headache, magnetic resonance imaging (MRI) of the brain is recommended.

During menstruation, the overall frequency of cluster headache attacks tends to improve.[2] Although the prevalence of cluster headache during pregnancy is very low, occurring in less than 0.3% of pregnancies, the severe and disabling nature of this headache disorder does impact women's

TABLE 15.1 Primary Headache Disorders Other Than Migraines

	Tension Headache	Trigeminal Neuralgia	Trigeminal Autonomic Cephalgias[a]			
			Short-Lasting Unilateral Neuralgiform Headache Attacks	Paroxysmal Hemicrania	Cluster	Hemicrania Continua
Female:male ratio	1-3:1	2.3:1	1:1.5	2–3:1	1:3	2:1
Diagnostic features	Mild to moderate pain No significant associated symptoms	Unilateral, severe electrical pain in the trigeminal distribution May have neurovascular contact or changes seen in trigeminal nerve	Lasting 1–600 seconds Referred to as SUNCT if conjunctival injection and tearing are present Referred to as SUNA if only one of the above or neither symptom is present	Lasting 2–30 minutes	Lasting 15–180 minutes Pain often excruciating and agitating Circadian and circannual pattern present	Lasting >3 months Often experience a foreign body sensation and stabbing pain

(continued)

TABLE 15.1 **Continued**

| | Tension Headache | Trigeminal Neuralgia | Trigeminal Autonomic Cephalgias[a] | | | |
			Short-Lasting Unilateral Neuralgiform Headache Attacks	Paroxysmal Hemicrania	Cluster	Hemicrania Continua
Treatment considerations	Optimize nonpharmacologic options	Carbamazepine (first-line treatment) reduces estrogen levels	Lamotrigine (first-line treatment)	Indomethacin responsive During pregnancy, important to consider premature closure of ductus arteriosus, oligohydramnios, and renal failure	For acute treatment, therapies should have rapid onset	Indomethacin responsive During pregnancy, important to consider premature closure of ductus arteriosus, oligohydramnios, and renal failure

[a]Class of unilateral head pain in the trigeminal nerve distribution, with associated autonomic symptoms ipsilateral to the side of pain.
SUNA, short-lasting unilateral neuralgiform headache attacks with cranial autonomic symptoms; SUNCT, short-lasting unilateral neuralgiform headache attacks with conjunctival injection and tearing.

> **BOX 15.1 Trigeminal Neuralgia**
>
> **Description**
>
> Attacks of severe, strictly unilateral pain that is orbital, supraorbital, temporal, or in any combination of these sites, lasting 15–180 minutes and occurring from once every other day to eight times a day. The pain is associated with ipsilateral conjunctival injection, lacrimation, nasal congestion, rhinorrhea, forehead and facial sweating, miosis, ptosis and/or eyelid edema, and/or with restlessness or agitation.
>
> **Diagnostic Criteria**
>
> A. At least five attacks fulfilling criteria B–D
> B. Severe or very severe unilateral orbital, supraorbital, and/or temporal pain lasting 15–180 minutes (when untreated)[1]
> C. Either or both of the following:
>   1. At least one of the following symptoms or signs, ipsilateral to the headache:
>   • Conjunctival injection and/or lacrimation
>   • Nasal congestion and/or rhinorrhea
>   • Eyelid edema
>   • Forehead and facial sweating
>   • Miosis and/or ptosis
>   2. A sense of restlessness or agitation
> D. Occurring with a frequency between 1 every other day and 8 per day[2]
> E. Not better accounted for by another *International Classification of Headache Disorders*, third edition (ICHD-3), diagnosis

decisions regarding family planning. Based on limited data, cluster headache may be unchanged or slightly improved during pregnancy, with an increased frequency of attacks postpartum.[2]

There are three types of treatments for cluster headache: acute treatments and transitional and maintenance therapy. For acute management, first-line treatment considered is oxygen inhalation, and fast-acting triptans such as intranasal or injectable formulations are preferred in light of the brief duration of cluster headache attacks.[3] Oxygen inhalation is a reasonable treatment option for pregnant patients, and triptans such as sumatriptan nasal spray may also be considered for pregnant patients.[2]

Corticosteroids are often used for transitional therapy; either a tapering course of oral corticosteroids or suboccipital corticosteroid injection (often with anesthetic) can be effective. It is advisable to consult with obstetrics before using corticosteroids during pregnancy. For preventative treatments, verapamil, lithium, topiramate, galcanezumab, and valproic acid can all be considered. Regarding safety in pregnancy, verapamil has not been shown to be associated with increased risk of fetal malformations, but one should be cautious that patients with cluster headaches may require higher doses than has been studied in pregnancy. Lithium, topiramate, and valproic acid are associated with increased risk of fetal and maternal complications and should be avoided in pregnancy. Very limited data on galcanezumab are available during pregnancy. As such, this medication should be avoided during pregnancy until more research is available. Invasive procedures such as occipital nerve stimulation and sphenopalatine ganglion stimulation could be considered.

Tension-Type Headaches

Tension headache is the most common primary headache syndrome, with a lifetime prevalence ranging from 30% to 78%.[1,4] In adults, there is an increased prevalence among females, ranging from 1.16 to 3 females for every 1 male.[4] Tension-type headache is characterized by mild to moderate pain without prominent associated symptoms. Diagnostic criteria are listed in Box 15.2.[1] The average age of patients is approximately 29 years.[5]

There is evidence that during menses, women experience an exacerbation of tension headaches either only during their menstrual cycle (28.5%) or during their menstrual cycle as well as other times in their cycle (71.5%).[5] Given the relatively mild nature of tension-type headache compared with migraine, behavioral strategies can be effective in treating tension-type headache. Acetaminophen may also be considered. To date, there is no evidence that treatment for tension-type headache should vary based on gender.

Little is known about the course of tension-type headache during pregnancy, with limited studies suggesting women with tension-type headache experience fewer changes during pregnancy than those with migraine.

> **BOX 15.2 Tension-Type Headache**
>
> **Diagnostic Criteria**
>
> A. At least 10 episodes of headache occurring on 1–14 days/month on average for >3 months (≥12 and <180 days/year) and fulfilling criteria B–D
> B. Lasting from 30 minutes to 7 days
> C. At least two of the following four characteristics:
>   1. Bilateral location
>   2. Pressing or tightening (non-pulsating) quality
>   3. Mild or moderate intensity
>   4. Not aggravated by routine physical activity such as walking or climbing stairs
> D. Both of the following:
>   1. No nausea or vomiting
>   2. No more than one of photophobia or phonophobia
> E. Not better accounted for by another ICHD-3 diagnosis

Trigeminal Neuralgia

Trigeminal neuralgia (TN) is unilateral, severe, electrical pain lasting from seconds to minutes.[1] It can be further divided into three categories based on the underlying etiology/lesions:

1. Idiopathic: No evidence of neurovascular contact or morphological changes of the trigeminal root
2. Classical: Evidence of neurovascular compression with morphological changes
3. Secondary: Due to a major neurological disease such as multiple sclerosis or a tumor

Patients can also be characterized by their presentation. Some have purely paroxysmal pain, whereas others experience concomitant continuous pain. The overall prevalence is approximately 70 per 100,000 individuals, and the incidence is 4.3–8 per 100,000 individuals.[6] It is more common in females, but this distribution changes after age 80 years, when TN becomes more common in males.[6]

When considering TN as a diagnosis, it is important to consider a broad differential for facial pain. The differential diagnostic considerations include herpes zoster, TACs, occipital or glossopharyngeal neuralgia, demyelinating disorders, temporomandibular joint pain, cerebral aneurysms, giant cell arteritis, tumors, intracranial hemorrhage, and recent dental procedure resulting in nerve injury. For young women, especially those with bilateral facial pain, multiple sclerosis should be considered, and further imaging, such as MRI, is warranted.

Based on limited data, TN is not expected to worsen in the setting of menstruation, pregnancy, or menopause.

First-line treatment for TN is carbamazepine. Other medications to consider include oxcarbazepine, lamotrigine, baclofen, gabapentin, pregabalin, phenytoin, amitriptyline, nortriptyline, and clonazepam.[7] Many of these medications have a teratogenic potential, rendering them inappropriate for use in pregnancy. Borrowing from epilepsy data, medications associated with lower risk of major congenital malformations include lamotrigine, which could be considered for treatment in patients with TN during pregnancy.[8] In addition, drug–drug interactions are an important consideration in particular for patients on estrogen-containing hormonal contraceptives or for patients undergoing gender-affirming hormone therapy. Carbamazepine and oxcarbazepine can reduce estrogen levels.[9] Patients refractory to medication, with clear evidence of vascular compression of the trigeminal nerve, may be candidates for surgical management, including microvascular decompression, percutaneous rhizotomy, and gamma knife radiosurgery.[7] Limited data also suggest that onabotulinum toxin A injections may be beneficial to treat TN. However, there is a lack of standardization among studies regarding the sites of onabotulinum toxin A injections and the dosage used. Another noninvasive approach to consider is peripheral nerve blocks without steroids.

KEY POINTS TO REMEMBER

- Cluster headache is three times more common in men than in women.
- Tension-type headache is the most common primary headache disorder, although the generally mild to moderate nature of the pain and responsiveness to over-the-counter analgesics render it a more manageable headache disorder compared with migraine.

References

1. Headache Classification Committee of the International Headache Society. *The international classification of headache disorders* (beta version). *Cephalalgia.* 2013;33(9):629–808.
2. van Vliet JA. Cluster headache in women: Relation with menstruation, use of oral contraceptives, pregnancy, and menopause. *J Neurol Neurosurg Psychiatry.* 2006;77:690–692.
3. Nahas SJ. Cluster headache and other trigeminal autonomic cephalalgias. *Continuum.* 2021;27:633–651.
4. Crystal SC, Robbins MS. Epidemiology of tension-type headache. *Curr Pain Headache Rep.* 2010;14:449–454.
5. Arjona A, Rubi-Callejon J, Guardado-Santervas P, Serrano-Castro P, Olivares J. Menstrual tension-type headache: Evidence for its existence. *Headache.* 2007;47:100–103.
6. Maarbjerg S, Benoliel R. The changing face of trigeminal neuralgia: A narrative review. *Headache.* 2021;61:817–837.
7. Hranilovich JA, Kaiser EA, Pace A, Barber M, Ziplow J. Headache in transgender and gender-diverse patients: A narrative review. *Headache.* 2021;61:1040–1050.
8. Li Y, Meador KJ. Epilepsy and pregnancy. *Continuum.* 2022;28:34–54.
9. Jones MR, Urits I, Ehrhardt KP, et al. A comprehensive review of trigeminal neuralgia. *Curr Pain Headache Rep.* 2019;23:74.

16 A Woman With a Headache in the Second Trimester

Christina R. Catherine

A 27-year-old woman who is 28 weeks pregnant presents to the neurology clinic for new-onset headaches that have started in the past few weeks. Headaches are worst in the mornings and worsen with cough or Valsalva. They are usually holocephalic with frontal predominance and occasionally also associated with blurry vision but no other associated symptoms. She reports that she has gained almost 50 pounds since the beginning of pregnancy (current weight is 220 pounds). Neurological examination is unremarkable except for blurring of the optic disc margins bilaterally (suggesting optic disc edema). Vitals show heart rate 95 beats per minute and blood pressure 111/67 mm Hg. She has trace, nonpitting peripheral edema mainly in bilateral lower extremities. Basic lab work with complete blood counts, basic metabolic panel, and urine protein:creatinine ratio was within normal limits.

What do you do now?

IDIOPATHIC INTRACRANIAL HYPERTENSION

New-onset headache in the second and third trimester may alert providers to possible hypertensive disorders of pregnancy; however, this patient has normal blood pressure and no sign of end organ damage/proteinuria on basic testing. She does present with signs of elevated intracranial pressure (ICP) given her visual obscurations and new-onset, persistent headache of several weeks' duration. Urgent neuroimaging with an MRI brain and MR venogram (MRV) to rule out underlying mass lesion or cerebral venous sinus thrombosis (CVST) are indicated, respectively. These should be performed without contrast, if possible, given the potential unknown risk to the fetus of in utero gadolinium exposure. Lumbar puncture in the left lateral decubitus position with opening pressure should be obtained after imaging. Cerebrospinal fluid (CSF) studies for glucose, protein, cell counts, cytology, and infectious agents (viral, bacterial, and fungal) should be sent for. In this case, the patient had an unremarkable MRI brain/MRV aside from a partially empty sella (Figure 16.1). Her opening pressure was 35 cm CSF with normal cell counts, cytology, and infectious studies, confirming her diagnosis of idiopathic intracranial hypertension (IIH).

IIH is a rare headache disorder that occurs in 0.5–2 per 100,000 people and is more common in patients with obesity.[1] Various criteria for IIH exist

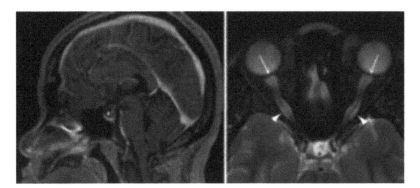

FIGURE 16.1 Brain MRI findings in IIH: Pictured on the left is a sagittal MRI showing an empty sella. The MRI on the right is an axial flair image showing tortuosity of the optic nerves with dilatation of the perioptic subarachnoid space.

(Box 16.1). Consensus criteria define IIH as a new or worsening headache associated with pulsatile tinnitus and/or optic disc edema, as well as elevated opening pressure when lumbar puncture is performed. There is ongoing debate regarding the exact pressure that constitutes elevated ICP, but opening pressures greater than 30 cm CSF have been suggested to be definitively abnormal. Opening pressures between 25 and 30 cm CSF are in a gray zone that may warrant further workup for both primary and secondary causes of elevated ICP.[1]

On examination, the patient may report transient visual obscurations, have unilateral or bilateral sixth nerve palsy, and have worsening of headache with Valsalva or when lying flat for extended periods of time. Neuroimaging

---

BOX 16.1 Idiopathic Intracranial Hypertension

The International Classification of Headache
***Disorders*, third edition (ICHD-3), Diagnostic Criteria**

A. New headache or significant worsening of a pre-existing headache fulfilling criteria C
B. Both of the following: IIH has been diagnosed and CSF pressure exceeds 25 cm CSF (or 28 cm CSF in obese children)
C. Either or both of the following are present:
   1. Headache developed or significantly worsened in temporal relation to IIH symptoms
   2. Headache is accompanied by either or both: pulsatile tinnitus or optic disc edema
D. Not better accounted for by another ICHD-3 diagnosis

Friedman Criteria for IIH

A. Optic disc edema present
B. Normal neurological examination (except for sixth cranial nerve palsy)
C. Neuroimaging: Normal brain parenchyma (no hydrocephalus, mass, structural lesion, or meningeal enhancement); venous thrombosis excluded
D. Normal CSF studies
E. Elevated opening pressure greater than 25 cm CSF
F. If optic disc edema is not present, can diagnose IIH if unilateral or bilateral sixth cranial nerve palsy present

should show normal brain parenchyma without evidence of hydrocephalus, mass lesion, cerebral venous sinus thrombosis, or external compression of the optic nerves. Imaging findings that may suggest elevated ICP include an empty sella, flattening of the posterior region of the globe, optic nerve tortuosity, and transverse sinus stenosis. CSF studies should show no signs of infection or malignancy.

Formal visual field testing by neuro-ophthalmology is preferred because vision loss is the main feared complication of IIH. Optical coherence tomography (OCT) and Humphrey visual field testing should be performed serially to monitor vision status until ICP normalizes.

Secondary causes of elevated ICP aside from CVST or mass lesion should also be considered in appropriate cases. In women of childbearing age or who are pregnant, the most common secondary causes to investigate include systemic lupus erythematosus, vitamin A/retinoid supplementation, lithium exposure, HIV, syphilis, Lyme disease, severe iron deficiency anemia, obstructive sleep apnea, hypoparathyroidism, and Turner syndrome.[1]

Treatment

First-line treatment of IIH during pregnancy includes weight control and medications. Moderate weight reduction (5–10%) is recommended prior to pregnancy if IIH diagnosis occurs prenatally. During pregnancy, consultation with a dietician should be sought to safely help maintain a safe weight because ketosis can have adverse fetal consequences. The use of acetazolamide during pregnancy is controversial because there are only limited safety data available. A small study of 101 women who took acetazolamide during pregnancy showed an increased rate of spontaneous and induced abortions in the acetazolamide group but no increased rates of malformations between the two groups.[1] In rodent studies, polydactyly and limb deficiency have been linked to perinatal acetazolamide exposure, but this link was not noted in primate studies. Topiramate and other diuretic medications that are sometimes given to patients with IIH are contraindicated during pregnancy given the much higher rate of congenital malformations that have been noted with these medications. Folic acid supplementation (>400 µg daily) should be recommended for all women trying to conceive and continued until at least the first trimester.[2]

Visual field testing should continue during pregnancy and be checked every 6–8 weeks with repeat OCT imaging and Humphrey visual field testing.[2] Treatment options should be adjusted depending on recurrence or worsening of visual symptoms after stabilization. If there is imminent risk to vision, serial high-volume lumbar punctures (LPs), optic nerve fenestration, or CSF diversion can be considered. Serial LPs can be repeated as needed for symptom control, especially for patients in the last trimester whose symptoms are likely to improve with the anticipated postpartum weight loss. None of these treatments have been shown to be significantly helpful in treating the headache of IIH and serve mainly to preserve vision.[1] European guidelines do not recommend CSF diversion/shunting techniques nor venous sinus stenting to treat headache symptoms given the risk of poor outcomes: ongoing headaches in 77% at 12 months post-shunting, high rates of necessary shunt revisions, or complications of stenting such as stent-adjacent stenosis that requires restenting in one-third of patients.[1] There are case reports of venous stenting being successful during pregnancy for fulminant IIH, but this should be approached on a case-by-case basis.[3]

Treatment of the headache of IIH should be based on the most closely related primary headache type (usually IIH headache is migrainous in nature). Prevention with lifestyle changes and medications if symptoms persist are indicated. Lifestyle changes, including adequate hydration (>2 liters daily during pregnancy), reduction in caffeine intake, adequate sleep, and mild to moderate daily exercise, should be encouraged. Some patients benefit from cognitive–behavioral therapy for management of their headaches, and referral to a female therapist trained in this area may be beneficial. Noninvasive devices using transmagnetic stimulation or trigeminal nerve stimulation may be beneficial, but these are still being researched. Low-dose acetaminophen, antiemetics, ibuprofen (if not in the third trimester), sumatriptan, or occipital nerve blocks are considered safe options for acute treatment of headaches. Preventative therapy is discussed elsewhere but can include magnesium supplementation, occipital nerve blocks, or prescription medications such as propranolol or tricyclic antidepressants after a personalized discussion on risks versus benefits is held.

Management During Labor and Birth

Idiopathic intracranial hypertension is not a medical indication for a termination or elective induction because gestation has not been shown to worsen IIH prognosis or affect perinatal outcome.[4] A recent retrospective chart review compared birth outcomes in women with or without IIH with primary outcomes of ectopic/molar pregnancy, abortion, preterm labor, preeclampsia/eclampsia, cesarean section, and maternal mortality.[5] There was no statistically significant difference between the two groups except for increased mortality in women with IIH (odds ratio: 5.279), although the reason for this increased mortality was not discussed in further detail. A recently published prospective cohort study (IIH Life) that included 377 patients showed that women with IIH diagnosis prior to pregnancy had no significant differences regarding visual or headache outcomes compared to women who did not have a pregnancy.[6] More severe papilledema was noted in women diagnosed with IIH during pregnancy, although diagnosis during pregnancy was a rare event, and long-term visual outcomes were comparable between all group participants regardless of pregnancy status.

Women with IIH can have neuraxial anesthesia during labor if desired. Both spinal and epidural anesthesia have been shown to be safe for these women.[1,2,4] Mode of delivery should be decided by obstetric factors only; normal vaginal delivery poses minimal risk to women with IIH, whereas cesarean section carries increased intrapartum and postoperative risks to the mother.[2] General anesthesia should be avoided if possible given increased risks, particularly to a patient with IIH because intubation, depth of anesthesia, and extubation are all associated with increased ICP.[4] If general anesthesia is required, propofol is the preferred induction agent because it decreases cerebral blood flow and thus ICP.[4] Succinylcholine should be avoided because muscle fasciculations can hypothetically elevate ICP.

KEY POINTS TO REMEMBER

- To establish the diagnosis of IIH requires that other secondary causes of elevated intracranial pressure be excluded, such as mass lesions and cerebral venous thrombosis. This is accomplished with MRI.

- Lumbar puncture is necessary to make the diagnosis and must show normal CSF contents with an opening pressure >25–30 cm CSF to confirm diagnosis.
- The major complication of IIH is visual loss, so a neuro-ophthalmology evaluation is important. Serial visual field testing should occur every 6–8 weeks during pregnancy.
- Management of IIH during pregnancy involves weight control and acetazolamide. Invasive procedures such as serial LP, stenting, or shunt placement can be considered on a case-by-case basis depending on severity of papilledema.
- The mode of delivery should be dictated by obstetric reasons. Normal vaginal delivery with neuraxial anesthesia per patient request is safe for women with IIH.

References

1. Hoffmann J, Mollan SP, Paemeleire K, et al. European Headache Federation guidelines on idiopathic intracranial hypertension. *J Headache Pain*. 2018;19:93. https://doi.org/10.1186/s10194-018-0919-2
2. Thaller M, Wakerley BR, Abbott S, Tahrani AA, Mollan SP, Sinclair AJ. Managing idiopathic intracranial hypertension in pregnancy: Practical advice. *Pract Neurol*. 2022;22:295–300.
3. Kamdar J, Gullo T, Strohm T. Idiopathic intracranial hypertension in a pregnant female improved with venous sinus stenting. *Neurology*. 2021;96(15 Suppl):4990.
4. Alves S, Sousa N, Cardoso L, Alves J. Multidisciplinary management of idiopathic intracranial hypertension in pregnancy: Case series and narrative review. *Braz J Anesthesiol*. 2022;72(6):790–794. https://doi.org/10.1016/j.bjane.2021.02.030
5. Hallan DR, Lin AC, Tankam CS, et al. Pregnancy and childbirth in women with idiopathic intracranial hypertension. *Cureus*. 2022;14(10):e30420. doi:10.7759/cureus.30420
6. Thaller M, Homer V, Mollan SP, Sinclair AJ. Disease course and long-term outcomes in pregnant women with idiopathic intracranial hypertension: The IIH Prospective Maternal Health Study. *Neurology*. 2023;100:e1598–e1610.

17 Acute Headache in Pregnancy

M. Angela O'Neal and Addie Peretz

A 27-year-old female who is currently 29 weeks pregnant is referred for evaluation of an acute headache for 9 days. She has a prior history of migraines. These new headaches have worsened over the course of a number of days and are refractory to treatment. Her headache continues to be debilitating. Imaging of the brain with magnetic resonance imaging (MRI) and MR venogram were obtained, which showed a pituitary lesion. She then woke up with a severe 10/10 headache and came to the emergency room with her husband. A repeat brain MRI was obtained (Figure 17.1).

What do you do now?

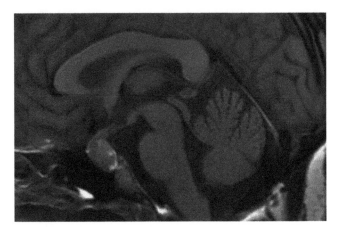

FIGURE 17.1 Sagittal T1 Brain MRI: Expanded pituitary with inhomogeneous intensity within the pituitary. Extension into the suprasellar cistern with compression of optic chiasm.

PITUITARY APOPLEXY

Definition

Pituitary apoplexy is a rare but potentially life-threatening disorder caused by hemorrhage or infarction of the pituitary gland. It occurs more commonly among patients with a pre-existing history of pituitary adenoma, affecting 0.2–0.6% of the general population and 2–12% of patients with pituitary adenomas.[1] Pituitary adenomas larger than 10 cm and rapidly growing tumors may be at higher risk for apoplexy. A number of medications or situations can predispose a patient to pituitary apoplexy, including endocrine stimulation tests, bromocriptine or cabergoline treatment, gonadotropin-releasing hormone treatment, lumbar fusion in the prone position, pregnancy, pituitary irradiation, anticoagulation, thrombocytopenia, and medications for erectile dysfunction. Pituitary apoplexy is a medical and in some cases surgical emergency that necessitates prompt evaluation and management.

Sheehan syndrome occurs in postpartum women and is characterized by pituitary ischemia and subsequent necrosis as a result of excessive bleeding during childbirth. Women suffering from Sheehan syndrome experience adrenal insufficiency, hypothyroidism, hypopituitarism, and, occasionally, visual changes.[2]

Anatomy

The pituitary gland sits at the base of the skull in the sella turcica and is divided into the anterior pituitary and posterior pituitary. The anterior pituitary receives blood from the hypothalamus along the infundibulum as venous channels connecting two capillary beds, the so-called portal system. The superior hypophyseal arteries give off branches that supply part of the infundibulum, which receives axons from numerous hypothalamic nuclei. These axons release various releasing and inhibiting factors, which are then taken down the infundibulum via the portal venous plexus and are delivered to the anterior pituitary, where they control the release of hormones. The posterior pituitary receives a rich network of arterial supply from the cavernous portion of the internal carotid artery. Due to this unique circulation, pituitary apoplexy can occur in certain circumstances.[3]

The mechanisms postulated for pituitary apoplexy include a rapidly growing adenoma that outstrips its blood supply. Alternatively, the enlarging mass may compress the portal veins, causing hemorrhagic necrosis. Other risk factors that are associated with pituitary apoplexy include acute changes in blood pressure, stimulation of the gland by increased estrogen states, and hormonal changes such as pregnancy and coagulopathy. Our patient had a macroadenoma that was rapidly expanding due the hormonal changes associated with pregnancy.[4]

Clinical Features

Pituitary apoplexy can present with a constellation of symptoms, most often visual disturbances, endocrine abnormalities, and headache. Headache is the most commonly reported symptom and can be sudden in onset and severe. Hypopituitarism can be characterized by Addisonian crisis and hyponatremia. With regard to visual disturbances, patients may experience reduced visual acuity, visual field disruption, and diplopia. Approximately 20% of patients will have a change in mental status from a mild encephalopathy to coma. Cranial nerve involvement can commonly occur, related to expansion into the cavernous sinus.

Endocrine Dysfunction

Pituitary apoplexy is a neuroendocrine emergency due to hormonal insufficiency. The lack of secretion of adrenocorticotropic hormone is most problematic and can cause adrenal crisis, with symptoms including nausea, vomiting, abdominal pain, bradycardia, hypotension, hypothermia, lethargy, and possibly coma. Other hormonal deficiencies in pituitary apoplexy include growth hormone, hypothyroidism, and hypogonadotropic deficiency. High prolactin levels may reflect a prolactinoma or be due to hypothalamic inhibition. Diabetes insipidus (DI) is also common.

Treatment

The most urgent issue is prompt assessment of fluid and electrolyte imbalance and replacement of corticosteroids. Acute adrenal insufficiency is seen in two-thirds of patients with pituitary apoplexy and is an important contributor to mortality. The role of surgery versus medical management is controversial.[5] Most agree that surgery is indicated when there is significant neurological impairment.

Our patient was admitted to the neurointensive care unit. She received 100 mg of hydrocortisone immediately and 2.5 mg of bromocriptine. Two days later, she woke with a severe headache, and her visual fields were constricted. After consultation with obstetric–anesthesia and maternal fetal medicine teams, she was taken to the operating room.

Her postoperative course was notable for the fact that she developed DI, complicating her management. She left the hospital to go home 9 days after admission. Two months later, she delivered a healthy baby boy.

KEY POINTS TO REMEMBER

- Pituitary apoplexy is a neurological emergency.
- The unique vasculature of the pituitary gland makes it vulnerable in certain circumstances to hemorrhage or infarction.
- The neuroendocrine status needs to be assessed immediately.
- Headaches, visual disturbance, and cranial neuropathies involving the nerves in the cavernous sinus are common presenting features.

References

1. Barkhoudarian G, Kelly DF. Pituitary apoplexy. *Neurosurg Clin North Am.* 2019;30:457–463.
2. Mayol Del Valle M, De Jesus O. *Pituitary apoplexy.* In: *StatPearls.* StatPearls Publishing; 2023.
3. Ranabir S, Baruah MP. Pituitary apoplexy. *Indian J Endocrinol Metab.* 2011;15(Suppl 3):S188–S196.
4. Vargas G, Gonzalez B, Guinto G, et al. Pituitary apoplexy in nonfunctioning pituitary macroadenomas: A case–control study. *Endocr Pract.* 2014;20:1274–1280.
5. Capatina C, Inder W, Karavitaki N, Wass JAH. Management of endocrine disease: Pituitary tumour apoplexy. *Eur J Endocrinol.* 2015;172:R179–R190.

18 Chiari Malformation in Pregnancy

Janet F. R. Waters

A 29-year-old female at 38 weeks of gestation presented to the emergency room with complaint of headache of 12 hours duration. The headache was right-sided, retro-orbital with throbbing quality. She was experiencing photophobia, phonophobia, and osmophobia. She had nausea but no emesis, and she noted no visual symptoms. Headache did not worsen with coughing or Valsalva. She had a history of migraines with similar symptoms in the past. She had never undergone imaging. Blood pressure was normal. She had no fever or neck stiffness. Neurologic exam was normal, including reflexes. She underwent non-contrast magnetic resonance venography to rule out venous sinus thrombosis, which was normal. Magnetic resonance imaging (MRI) revealed Chiari I malformation with descent of the cerebellar tonsils 8 mm below the foramen magnum. Her obstetrician consulted neurology to ask if this patient could safely undergo vaginal delivery and epidural or spinal anesthesia.

What do you do now?

CHIARI MALFORMATIONS

Chiari malformations (types I–IV) are a group of congenital posterior fossa abnormalities that affect the structural relationships between the bony cranial base, cerebellum, brainstem, and cervical spinal cord.[1] Chiari I is defined as a descent of the cerebellar tonsils below the foramen magnum by 5 mm or more. In some individuals, it may be associated with cervical syringomyelia. In patients with Chiari II, both the cerebellum and brainstem tissue protrude into the foramen magnum. The malformation may be accompanied by a myelomeningocele—a form of spina bifida that occurs when the spinal canal and backbone do not fully close during development. In Chiari III, there is herniation of the cerebellum with or without the brainstem through a posterior encephalocele. Chiari IV malformation is defined as cerebellar hypoplasia or aplasia with a normal posterior fossa without hindbrain herniation. Chiari III and IV malformations are rare and usually not compatible with survival.

Chiari I malformations are common and can be found in 0.6% of the population. Patients with Chiari I are frequently asymptomatic but may present with a constellation of symptoms, including headaches that are exacerbated by coughing, Valsalva, or positional changes. More severely affected patients may present with cerebellar symptoms, quadriparesis, lower cranial nerve palsies, as well as central cord signs. As the utilization of brain imaging has become more common, Chiari I malformations are more frequently discovered, often as an incidental finding.

In the past, pregnant women with Chiari I malformation were considered to be high-risk patients by their obstetricians due to concerns of increasing intracranial pressure during active labor. It was not uncommon for these patients to be delivered by cesarean section to avoid the potential risk of elevated intracranial pressure. In addition, obstetrical anesthesiologists were reluctant to offer neuraxial anesthesia to women with Chiari I malformation due to concerns for changes in pressure gradients associated with inadvertent dural puncture.

Case reports and retrospective studies have not supported these concerns.[2,3] The safety of vaginal delivery and neuraxial anesthesia in women who have been decompressed has been well documented. A number of case reports have noted that asymptomatic patients with Chiari I malformation could also safely undergo vaginal delivery and spinal or epidural anesthesia.[4] A retrospective study done in 2018 confirmed the absence of neurologic complications in 97 deliveries of women with Chiari I malformation regardless of mode of delivery or anesthetic management.[5] The authors concluded that in women with Chiari I malformation without symptoms of increased intracranial pressure, mode of delivery should be based on obstetrical considerations. In addition, women with Chiari I malformation appeared to be at no higher risk of neurologic complication from neuraxial anesthesia than the general population.

The patient described in this chapter presented with findings suggestive of a recurrence of her migraine headache. Her headache had migrainous features and was not associated with Valsalva or cough. Her neurologic exam was normal. The Chiari malformation noted on her MRI was an incidental finding. Her headache can be managed with hydration and a modified migraine cocktail including an anti-nausea agent, acetaminophen, and diphenhydramine. Mode of delivery may be based on obstetrical considerations. There is no neurologic contraindication to epidural or spinal anesthesia.

KEY POINTS TO REMEMBER

- In patients who have asymptomatic Chiari I malformation, mode of delivery should be based on obstetric rather than neurologic considerations.
- In symptomatic patients, an obstetrical plan should be developed on an individual basis.
- The absence of complications in patients who received epidural or spinal anesthesia suggests that these agents should be made available to women with Chiari I malformation.

References

1. Ropper AH, Samuels, MA, Klein, JP. Developmental diseases of the nervous system. In: Sydor AM, Davis KJ, eds. *Adams and Victor's Principles of Neurology*. 10th ed. McGraw Hill; 2014:1015–1017.
2. Mueller DM, Oro' J. Chiari I malformation with or without syringomyelia and pregnancy: Case studies and review of the literature. *Am J Perinatol*. 2005;22(2):67–70. doi:10.1055/s-2005-837271

3. Roper JC, Al Wattar BH, Silva AHD, Samarasekera S, Flint G, Pirie AM. Management and birth outcomes of pregnant women with Chiari malformations: A 14 years retrospective case series. *Eur J Obstet Gynecol Reprod Biol*. 2018;230:1–5. doi:10.1016/j.ejogrb.2018.09.006

4. Sastry R, Sufianov R, Laviv Y, et al. Chiari I malformation and pregnancy: A comprehensive review of the literature to address common questions and to guide management. *Acta Neurochir*. 2020;162(7):1565–1573. doi:10.1007/s00701-020-04308-7

5. Waters JFR, O'Neal MA, Pilato M, Waters S, Larkin JC, Waters JH. Management of anesthesia and delivery in women with Chiari I malformations. *Obstet Gynecol*. 2018;132(5):1180–1184. doi:10.1097/AOG.0000000000002943

19 The Worst Headache of Her Life

Alison Seitz and Eliza Miller

A 34-year-old woman G3 P2 at 28 weeks of gestation reported sudden onset of the worst headache of her life. En route to the hospital, she became obtunded, arousable only to painful stimulation. On arrival, her blood pressure was 160/90 mm Hg. In the emergency room, she had two generalized tonic–clonic seizures. She was noted to have anisocoria: The left pupil was 5 mm and the right 2 mm. Only the right pupil reacted to light. Oculocephalic and corneal responses were present. She had decerebrate posturing. Head computed tomography (CT) scan was obtained and is shown in Figure 19.1, in addition to CT angiogram and CT venogram.

What do you do now?

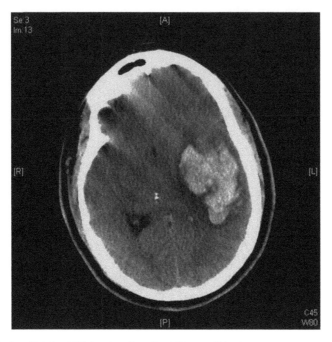

FIGURE 19.1 Plain head CT showing a large frontal temporal bleed.

ARTERIOVENOUS MALFORMATION

This case is an example of a ruptured arteriovenous malformation (AVM) causing an intracerebral hemorrhage during pregnancy. Volume changes that occur during pregnancy may increase the risk of AVM rupture. Once there has been a hemorrhage related to an AVM, the risk of re-rupture is high. Treatment of a ruptured AVM is dictated by best neurosurgical considerations because this condition is life-threatening. If needed, an emergent cesarean section and neurosurgical procedure can be done in tandem.

Unruptured AVM

Some studies report an increased risk of AVM rupture during pregnancy,[1–3] but some do not.[4] Many patients with unruptured AVMs can tolerate a vaginal delivery.[5,6] There are no data on the best management of unruptured AVMs during pregnancy, and outside of the setting of pregnancy, the data are similarly inconclusive.[7] If treatment of an asymptomatic, unruptured AVM is planned, this should be done prior to pregnancy.

Ruptured AVM

Once there has been a hemorrhage related to an AVM before or during pregnancy, the risk of rebleeding is high.[1] Treatment should be dictated by neurosurgical considerations rather than obstetric concerns because a ruptured AVM is life-threatening. Our patient was intubated and underwent an emergency cesarean section and craniotomy with clot evacuation and resection of the AVM, done in tandem. The next day, to ensure complete resection of the vascular lesion, she underwent cerebral angiography, which showed a small AVM with an intranidal aneurysm (Figure 19.2). She then underwent definitive resection of the AVM.

Intracerebral Hemorrhage

Most cases of intracerebral hemorrhage (ICH) in pregnancy occur as complications of hypertensive disorders of pregnancy (covered elsewhere in this textbook). Some, like our patient's ICH, are due to preexisting vascular lesions, such as AVMs, aneurysms, cavernous malformations, or fragile moyamoya collaterals. Any pregnant or postpartum patient with ICH, including from a ruptured AVM, should be transferred to a neurological intensive care unit and treated with blood pressure control, reversal of any coagulopathy, and, in the event of life-threatening mass effect, hematoma

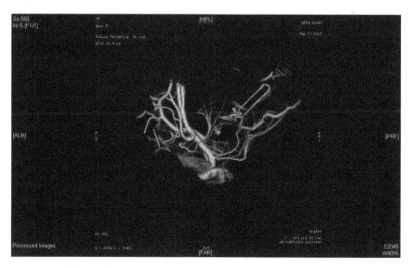

FIGURE 19.2 The arteriogram shows the vascular malformation with a nidal aneurysm.

evacuation.[7] Patients with ruptured AVMs treated in dedicated neurological intensive care units can have good long-term maternal and fetal outcomes.[8]

> **KEY POINTS TO REMEMBER**
>
> - Treatment of a ruptured AVM is based on best neurosurgical practice. If delivery of the fetus is needed, this can be done in tandem with neurosurgical treatment.
> - Any pregnant or postpartum patient with ICH should be transferred to a neurosurgical intensive care unit.
> - If treatment of an unruptured AVM is planned, it should be done prior to pregnancy.

References

1. Porras JL, Yang W, Philadelphia E, et al. Hemorrhage risk of brain arteriovenous malformations during pregnancy and puerperium in a North American cohort. *Stroke*. 2017;48:1507–1513.
2. Lee S, Kim Y, Navi BB, et al. Risk of intracranial hemorrhage associated with pregnancy in women with cerebral arteriovenous malformations. *J Neurointerv Surg*. 2021;13:707–710.
3. Liu J, Zhang H, Luo C, et al. Haemorrhage risk of brain arteriovenous malformation during pregnancy and puerperium. *Stroke Vasc Neurol*. 2023;8(4):307–317.
4. Liu X, Wang S, Zhao Y, et al. Risk of cerebral arteriovenous malformation rupture during pregnancy and puerperium. *Neurology*. 2014;82:1798–1803.
5. Katsuragi S, Yoshimatsu J, Tanaka H, et al. Management of pregnancy complicated with intracranial arteriovenous malformation. *J Obstet Gynaecol Res*. 2018;44:673–680.
6. Lv X, Li W, He H, Jiang C, Li Y. Known and unknown cerebral arteriovenous malformations in pregnancies: Haemorrhage risk and influence on obstetric management. *Neuroradiol J*. 2017;30:437–441.
7. Derdeyn CP, Zipfel GJ, Albuquerque FC, et al. Management of brain arteriovenous malformations: A scientific statement for healthcare professionals from the American Heart Association/American Stroke Association. *Stroke*. 2017;48:e200–e224.
8. Yan KL, Ko NU, Hetts SW, et al. Maternal and fetal outcomes in women with brain arteriovenous malformation rupture during pregnancy. *Cerebrovasc Dis*. 2021;50:296–302.

20 Postpartum Left-Sided Numbness and Right-Sided Shaking

Alison Seitz and Eliza Miller

A 20-year-old woman 10 days postpartum from an uncomplicated cesarean section for which she had spinal anesthesia presented with a diffuse headache. The prior day, she noted left-sided numbness. The day of admission, she had right arm shaking followed by a generalized tonic–clonic seizure. Her blood pressure was 110/70 mm Hg and temperature was 97.8°F. She was drowsy and inattentive but otherwise had no focal deficits on examination.

What do you do now?

CEREBRAL VENOUS THROMBOSIS

Incidence and Pathophysiology

Cerebral venous thrombosis (CVT) accounts for approximately one-third of pregnancy-related strokes, with an incidence of approximately 9.1 per 100,000 deliveries.[1] Most cases occur postpartum.[2] Pregnant patients are most hypercoagulable in the third trimester and first 6 weeks postpartum.[3,4] Patients with cesarean delivery, hypertension, and infections other than pneumonia and influenza,[5] and possibly those who experienced dural puncture,[6] are at higher risk of CVT (Figure 20.1).

Clinical Features

Cerebral venous thrombosis presents with headache from elevated intracranial pressure in 70–90% of patients. Patients commonly develop focal neurologic syndromes from hemorrhage or venous infarcts that generally do not respect arterial territories, and many develop seizures. In our

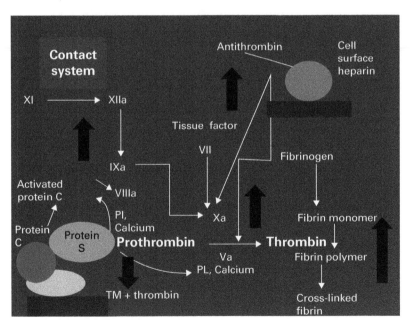

FIGURE 20.1 Depicted are the major changes in clotting factors that occur in pregnancy, ultimately leading to an increase in thrombin production and decreased thrombolytic activity.

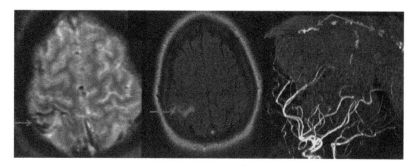

FIGURE 20.2 The image on the left is a gradient echo sequence showing susceptibility in the right parietal sulci. The middle image is the fluid-attenuated inversion recovery sequence showing hyperintensity in the same location. These are due to a right parietal vein thrombosis. The image on the right is a brain MRA showing areas of high signal at the superior aspect of the sagittal sinus, consistent with thrombosis.

patient, a brain MRI, MR arteriogram, and MR venogram confirmed the diagnosis (Figure 20.2).

Treatment

Patients with CVT are at high risk for clinical deterioration, including progression of edema, hemorrhage, increased intracranial pressure, and herniation, and must be monitored closely. The treatment for CVT is anticoagulation, even in the presence of hemorrhage. Heparin and its derivatives do not cross the placenta and can be used during pregnancy.[7] A hypercoagulability workup should be completed, although some markers may be falsely elevated during pregnancy. If negative, anticoagulation can be discontinued after 3–12 months or after recanalization.[8] Hematology consultation is recommended. Seizures are treated with standard anticonvulsants. Prophylactic use of anticonvulsants is not routinely recommended.[8]

In our patient, a full hypercoagulability evaluation was done and unremarkable. She started treatment with heparin with a plan to transition to warfarin, which is safe during lactation, for 6 months.

Future Pregnancies

Cerebral venous thrombosis is not a contraindication for future pregnancies, but patients with a history of CVT may benefit from prophylactic anticoagulation with low-molecular-weight heparin in future pregnancies and up to 12 weeks postpartum.

KEY POINTS TO REMEMBER

- CVT can present with headache, focal neurologic syndromes from venous infarcts or hemorrhage, and seizures.
- Hematological changes that occur in pregnancy result in a hypercoagulable state which predispose to CVT.
- CVT is treated with anticoagulation.
- Anticoagulation is recommended for future pregnancies.

References

1. Swartz RH, Cayley ML, Foley N, et al. The incidence of pregnancy-related stroke: A systematic review and meta-analysis. *Int J Stroke*. 2017;12:687–697.
2. Silvis SM, Lindgren E, Hiltunen S, et al. Postpartum period is a risk factor for cerebral venous thrombosis. *Stroke*. 2019;50:501–503.
3. Kamel H, Navi BB, Sriram N, Hovsepian DA, Devereux RB, Elkind MSV. Risk of a thrombotic event after the 6-week postpartum period. *N Engl J Med*. 2014;370:1307–1315.
4. Clark P, Brennand J, Conkie JA, McCall F, Greer IA, Walker ID. Activated protein C sensitivity, protein C, protein S and coagulation in normal pregnancy. *Thromb Haemost*. 1998;79:1166–1170.
5. Lanska DJ, Kryscio RJ. Risk factors for peripartum and postpartum stroke and intracranial venous thrombosis. *Stroke*. 2000;31:1274–1282.
6. Chambers DJ, Bhatia K, Columb M. Postpartum cerebral venous sinus thrombosis following obstetric neuraxial blockade: A literature review with analysis of 58 case reports. *Int J Obstet Anesth*. 2022;49:103218.
7. Algahtani H, Bazaid A, Shirah B, Bouges RN. Cerebral venous sinus thrombosis in pregnancy and puerperium: A comprehensive review. *Brain Circ*. 2022;8:180–187.
8. Ropper AH, Klein JP. Cerebral venous thrombosis. *N Engl J Med*. 2021;385:59–64.

SECTION IV

Stroke and Vascular Disorders

21 A Pregnant Woman With Aphasia and Right-Sided Weakness

Alison Seitz and Eliza Miller

A 28-year-old woman, G2 P1 at 30 weeks gestation, was last seen well at 10 a.m. Fifty minutes later, she was found on the ground, not speaking or moving her right side. On arrival to the emergency department, her blood pressure was 130/80 mm Hg. She was mute, with left gaze deviation and right hemiplegia. Her noncontrast head computed tomography (CT) scan was normal.

What do you do now?

ISCHEMIC STROKE

Incidence and Etiology of Ischemic Stroke

In pregnancy, the incidence of all stroke is approximately 30 per 100,000 deliveries, and the incidence of ischemic stroke is approximately 12.2 per 100,000 deliveries.[1] The highest risk of maternal stroke occurs in the peripartum and immediate postpartum period,[1] but it remains elevated until at least 12 weeks after delivery[2] and possibly until 1 year postpartum. Risk factors include older age, migraine, underlying prothrombotic conditions, inflammatory disorders such as systemic lupus erythematosus, connective tissue disorders, heart disease, hypertensive disorders of pregnancy, and postpartum hemorrhage or infection.[3] Social determinants of health significantly impact stroke risk such that Black pregnant and postpartum patients have disproportionately high rates of stroke and mortality regardless of socioeconomic status and medical comorbidities.[4]

Physiologic changes in pregnancy increase the risk of stroke. Cardiac output and systemic vasodilation increase, leading to greater risk of arrhythmias and venous thromboembolism. Pregnant patients are also hypercoagulable and have a physiologic dilutional anemia. Arterial ischemic stroke, as in our patient, can occur due to paradoxical embolism; heart disease; cervical or intracranial artery dissection; reversible cerebral vasoconstriction syndrome; ovarian hyperstimulation syndrome; hypercoagulability; or hemolysis, elevated liver enzymes, and low platelet syndrome complicated by disseminated intravascular coagulation; in addition to rarer causes.

Treatment

Imaging should not be delayed due to pregnancy when acute ischemic stroke is suspected. The dose of ionizing radiation from a noncontrast CT head is below the threshold above which adverse fetal effects are seen, and although the contrast from CT angiography confers a theoretical (never demonstrated in human studies) risk of neonatal hypothyroidism, the benefit of CT angiography for rapid diagnosis of an acute large vessel occlusion

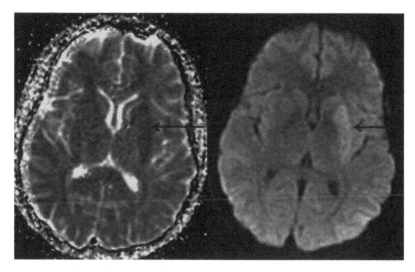

FIGURE 21.1 Brain MRI apparent diffusion coefficient imaging on the left and diffusion-weighted imaging on the right showing an acute infarct in the lenticulostriate territory.

outweighs the risk.[5] Magnetic resonance imaging (MRI) with MR angiography (MRA) is a reasonable alternative if it can be obtained immediately. Gadolinium should be avoided.

Pregnant patients with acute ischemic stroke can be treated with IV thrombolysis in addition to thrombectomy (with abdominal shielding) using the same guidelines as those for nonpregnant patients.[5-8] There is less evidence for the use of thrombolysis in the immediate postpartum period, but it may be considered.[6] A high-risk obstetrician and, if available, an obstetric anesthesiologist should be involved in all decisions regarding thrombolysis and mechanical thrombectomy.

Our patient received IV thrombolysis. Brain MRI and MRA of the head and neck images are shown in Figures 21.1 and 21.2. Her weakness and aphasia did not improve after IV thrombolysis, but she subsequently underwent mechanical thrombectomy and recovered with mild deficits.[8]

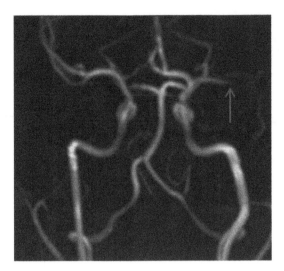

FIGURE 21.2 Brain MRA showing the occlusion of the left middle cerebral artery.

> **KEY POINTS TO REMEMBER**
> - Ischemic stroke in pregnancy is a rare but substantial cause of morbidity.
> - The causes of ischemic stroke in pregnancy are diverse.
> - Stroke characteristics should guide treatment in consultation with the obstetrical team.

References
1. Swartz RH, Cayley ML, Foley N, et al. The incidence of pregnancy-related stroke: A systematic review and meta-analysis. *Int J Stroke.* 2017;12:687–697.
2. Kamel H, Navi BB, Sriram N, Hovsepian DA, Devereux RB, Elkind MSV. Risk of a thrombotic event after the 6-week postpartum period. *N Engl J Med.* 2014;370:1307–1315.
3. James AH, Bushnell CD, Jamison MG, Myers ER. Incidence and risk factors for stroke in pregnancy and the puerperium. *Obstet Gynecol.* 2005;106:509–516.
4. Elgendy IY, Gad MM, Mahmoud AN, Keeley EC, Pepine CJ. Acute stroke during pregnancy and puerperium. *J Am Coll Cardiol.* 2020;75:180–190.
5. Ladhani NNN, Swartz RH, Foley N, et al. Canadian Stroke Best Practice Consensus Statement: Acute stroke management during pregnancy. *Int J Stroke.* 2018;13:743–758.

6. Powers WJ, Rabinstein AA, Ackerson T, et al. Guidelines for the early management of patients with acute ischemic stroke: 2019 update to the 2018 guidelines for the early management of acute ischemic stroke: A guideline for healthcare professionals from the American Heart Association/American Stroke Association. *Stroke*. 2019;50:e344–e418.
7. Leffert LR, Clancy CR, Bateman BT, et al. Treatment patterns and short-term outcomes in ischemic stroke in pregnancy or postpartum period. *Am J Obstet Gynecol*. 2016;214:723.e1–723.e11.
8. Dicpinigaitis AJ, Sursal T, Morse CA, et al. Endovascular thrombectomy for treatment of acute ischemic stroke during pregnancy and the early postpartum period. *Stroke*. 2021;52(12):3796–3804.

22 "Will I Have a Stroke?"

Alison Seitz and Eliza Miller

A 46-year-old woman with a history of prediabetes and stage 1 hypertension is referred for evaluation of her stroke risk. She does not smoke and drinks one or two alcoholic beverages a week. She has never had a transient ischemic attack or stroke. She had a twin pregnancy at age 28 years complicated by preeclampsia. Her exam is normal.

What do you do now?

STROKE

Incidence

Stroke is the third leading cause of death for women in the United States.[1] Average age at stroke is higher in women than men, with a significant increase in risk after menopause.[2] Sex-specific risk factors for stroke in women include pregnancy, adverse pregnancy outcomes, and estrogen-containing medications, and several other risk factors have a differential impact in women.

Risk Factors With a Differential Impact in Women

Some data show that diabetes, hypertension, and atrial fibrillation are more strongly associated with stroke risk in women than in men.[2] Elderly women with atrial fibrillation are at an especially high risk for subsequent stroke events. Migraine with aura is a risk factor for stroke, particularly in young adults; it has four times higher prevalence in women than men.[2]

Sex-Specific Risk Factors

Adverse pregnancy outcomes including gestational hypertension, preeclampsia, eclampsia, preterm birth, small-for-gestational-age infant, and placental abruption are associated with earlier onset of cerebrovascular disease.[3] Pregnancy itself is also a risk factor for stroke during pregnancy and up to 12 weeks postpartum.[4,5] Combined hormonal contraceptives are associated with increased stroke risk and merit a risk–benefit conversation in women with other stroke risk factors.[2] Postmenopausal estrogen-containing hormone therapy may increase the risk of stroke.[2,6]

Recommendations for Our Patient

Currently, optimal stroke risk management in women entails aggressive treatment of modifiable risk factors.[2] We discussed with our patient "Life's Essential 8": healthy diet; participation in physical activity; avoidance of nicotine; healthy sleep; healthy weight; and healthy levels of blood lipids, blood glucose, and blood pressure.[7] Our patient already avoids nicotine. We also discussed with her maintaining a healthy diet, weight, and sleep and participation in physical activity. She should proactively decrease her blood pressure and manage her blood sugar.

KEY POINTS TO REMEMBER

- Stroke is the third leading cause of death in women in the United States.
- Stroke risk factors that are unique to women include adverse pregnancy outcomes and estrogen-containing medications.
- Migraine with aura, atrial fibrillation, diabetes, high body mass index, and hypertension are stroke risk factors that have a greater impact in women than men.
- Risk mitigation entails aggressive management of modifiable risk factors.

References

1. Centers for Disease Control and Prevention. From CDC—Leading causes of death—Females all races and origins 2018 [online]. 2022. Accessed September 22, 2022. https://www.cdc.gov/women/lcod/2018/all-races-origins/index.htm
2. Bushnell C, McCullough LD, Awad IA, et al. Guidelines for the prevention of stroke in women. *Stroke*. 2014;45:1545–1588.
3. Miller EC, Kauko A, Tom SE, Laivuori H, Niiranen T, Bello NA. Risk of midlife stroke after adverse pregnancy outcomes: The FinnGen study. *Stroke*. 2023;54:1798–1895.
4. Swartz RH, Cayley ML, Foley N, et al. The incidence of pregnancy-related stroke: A systematic review and meta-analysis. *Int J Stroke*. 2017;12:687–697.
5. Kamel H, Navi BB, Sriram N, Hovsepian DA, Devereux RB, Elkind MSV. Risk of a thrombotic event after the 6-week postpartum period. *N Engl J Med*. 2014;370:1307–1315.
6. Marjoribanks J, Farquhar CM, Roberts H, Lethaby A. Cochrane corner: Long-term hormone therapy for perimenopausal and postmenopausal women. *Heart*. 2018;104:93–95.
7. Lloyd-Jones DM, Allen NB, Anderson CA, et al. Life's essential 8: Updating and enhancing the American Heart Association's construct of cardiovascular health: A presidential advisory from the American Heart Association. *Circulation*. 2022;146:e18–e43.

SECTION V

Neuromuscular Disorders and Neuropathies

23 A Young Woman With Double Vision and Fatigue

Carolina Barnett-Tapia and Vera Bril

A 28-year-old female has developed double vision, which is worse at the end of the day, and generalized fatigue. On examination, there is mild bilateral ptosis, which worsens after looking up for a prolonged period. Her extraocular movements are normal, but she reports double vision when looking up and toward the left. She has normal voice and speech, but she has mild proximal muscle weakness in the upper and lower extremities, which worsens with repetitive testing. Acetylcholine receptor antibodies are positive. Contrast computed tomography (CT) of the chest was planned to assess for thymoma, but a pregnancy test administered prior to CT was positive.

What do you do now?

MYASTHENIA GRAVIS AND PREGNANCY

Myasthenia gravis (MG) is a chronic autoimmune disorder caused by antibodies against the postsynaptic neuromuscular junction. Patients with MG typically experience fluctuating weakness in striated muscles, and they can present with ptosis, diplopia, dysphagia, dysarthria, and proximal limb weakness and combinations of these. In severe cases, there can be respiratory failure needing assisted ventilation. Diagnosis is usually based on positive antibodies against the acetylcholine receptor in 80–90% and against muscle-specific kinase (MuSK) antibody in approximately 10%; some patients can be seronegative. Thymoma is found in approximately 15% of individuals with MG, but it is more common in older patients.[1]

The estimated prevalence of MG is approximately 30 per 100,000 individuals, with a bimodal distribution and with a peak in young women and another in older men. Because of the peak in women of childbearing age, issues related to pregnancy and delivery are important for this group of patients. The relationship between MG and pregnancy is threefold and includes (1) the effects of pregnancy on MG, (2) the effects of MG on pregnancy outcomes, and (3) the effects of MG and its treatments in the fetus and newborn.[2]

The Effects of Pregnancy in Myasthenia Gravis

Several case series have found that in 30–60% of pregnancies there may be an exacerbation of myasthenic symptoms.[3,4] This usually occurs in the first trimester, last trimester, or during the postpartum period. Approximately one-third of women are stable and one-third have improvement of MG symptoms during pregnancy. In one case series, stopping or reducing the dose of treatments before or during pregnancy was associated with disease exacerbation and even crisis during pregnancy.[3] Some women may have a new onset of MG during pregnancy or in the postpartum period.

For women with a known diagnosis of MG, recommendations are to plan for pregnancy when the disease is stable. Many commonly used MG treatments, including pyridostigmine and prednisone, can be used in pregnancy and should be maintained unless there are major risks for an individual patient. Azathioprine, a commonly used steroid-sparing immunosuppressant in MG and multiple autoimmune diseases, is also considered low-risk in pregnancy, with data on hundreds of pregnancies showing no increased risk of congenital malformations. Tacrolimus is a calcineurin inhibitor that is also considered low risk for use in pregnancy and breastfeeding. Mycophenolate and methotrexate are teratogenic and should be avoided in women planning a pregnancy. Intravenous immunoglobulins (IVIG) and plasma exchange are low risk in pregnancy and can be used to treat exacerbations including crisis. IVIG or subcutaneous immunoglobulins can also be used as maintenance treatment during pregnancy if needed—for example, if a contraindicated treatment has to be stopped.[2,5]

If a patient is receiving a medication absolutely contraindicated in pregnancy, such as methotrexate or mycophenolate, it is recommended to change treatment at least 3 months before conception. In the case of an unplanned pregnancy, sudden discontinuation carries risk of acute exacerbation and crisis, and thus, patients should be followed by a high-risk obstetrics clinic as well as a neurologist with experience with MG. Table 23.1 summarizes commonly used medications in MG and the relationship to pregnancy and breastfeeding.

TABLE 23.1 **Common Therapeutic Interventions in Myasthenia Gravis**

Intervention	Potential Side Effects	Use in Pregnancy	Use While Breastfeeding
Pyridostigmine	Diarrhea, muscle cramps, increased secretions	Low risk; continue at standard dose.	Compatible; continue at standard dose.
Prednisone	Weight gain, hyperglycemia, hypertension, mood changes, osteoporosis	Low risk; use at lowest effective dose. Monitor for diabetes and hypertension. May need stress dose at delivery.	Compatible; use at lowest effective dose.
Azathioprine	Hepatoxicity, bone marrow suppression, nausea, diarrhea	Low risk. No increased risk of congenital malformations or adverse pregnancy outcomes. Unclear association with smaller neonatal weight. Continue at standard dose.	Compatible; continue at standard dose.

(*Continued*)

TABLE 23.1 **Continued**

Intervention	Potential Side Effects	Use in Pregnancy	Use While Breastfeeding
Mycophenolate mofetil	Hepatoxicity, bone marrow suppression, nausea, diarrhea	High risk. Teratogenic (e.g., diaphragmatic hernia, micrognathia, cleft lip/palate, and congenital heart defects). Stop before pregnancy.	Unknown
Tacrolimus	Nephrotoxicity, bone marrow suppression, hypothyroidism, hyperglycemia, hyperkalemia	Low risk. No increased risk of congenital malformations Continue at standard dose. Monitor levels.	Compatible; continue at standard dose.
Methotrexate	Bone marrow suppression, hair loss	High risk. Teratogenic, increased risk of miscarriage. Stop before pregnancy.	Not compatible; do not use.
Plasma exchange	Paresthesia, rash, hypotension, hypofibrinogenemia, electrolyte imbalances, nausea, vomiting, sepsis, vascular access complications	Low risk Usually as rescue treatment in case of severe exacerbation/ crisis.	Compatible
Immunoglobulins	Headache, rash, fever, aseptic meningitis, allergic/ anaphylactic reactions, hypercoagulability, hemolytic anemia	Low risk Can be used intravenously as rescue treatment. Subcutaneous route can be used as maintenance treatment.	Compatible; use standard dose.

Adapted from Cahill AG, Porter TF[5]

Effects of Myasthenia Gravis in Pregnancy Outcomes

Multiple cohort studies have assessed whether MG confers higher risk of adverse pregnancy outcomes. One large study in Canada found no difference in rate of spontaneous abortion, stillbirths, preeclampsia, eclampsia, cesarean sections, or assisted delivery (e.g., vacuum and forceps) between women with MG and controls, but it did find a slight increase in peripartum hemorrhage.[6] A study in Taiwan did not find any significant difference in cesarean sections or preterm delivery between women with MG and controls.[7]

Although MG does not confer a higher risk of preeclampsia and eclampsia, management has special considerations in MG. The standard treatment for eclampsia and severe preeclampsia includes intravenous magnesium for preventing seizures. Magnesium blocks calcium from entering the nerve terminal and inhibits the release of acetylcholine. Thus, it can cause exacerbations of MG in some cases, leading to respiratory failure. Therefore, intravenous magnesium is contraindicated in myasthenia. Published case reports of preeclampsia and eclampsia in MG have suggested the use of phenytoin, diazepam, and levetiracetam to prevent seizures.[8] The latter may be preferred in pregnancy because it has few interactions, does not need monitoring of drug levels, and does not have increased teratogenic risk. Box 23.1 shows list of medications to be used with caution in MG.

BOX 23.1 **Medications Known to Exacerbate Symptoms of Myasthenia Gravis**

Marked Contraindication, Should Be Avoided

- Telithromycin, botulinum toxin, D-penicillamine, fluoroquinolones.
- Intravenous magnesium: Use only if absolutely necessary and monitor for worsening.

Relative Contraindication, Use With Caution

- Macrolide antibiotics: Use cautiously if at all.
- Aminoglycosides: Use cautiously if no other alternative available.
- Beta-blockers, including propranolol and atenolol: Use cautiously.
- Iodinated contrast agents (older reports); modern contrast agents appear safer: Use cautiously and observe for worsening.

MG itself is not an indication for cesarean section, and this should be reserved for obstetrical reasons. During delivery, medications should be given as per typical doses, with special focus on maintaining pyridostigmine dosing because this provides rapid symptomatic benefit but only lasts for approximately 4 hours. Women with chronic use of steroids may need a stress dose at delivery.

Effects of Myasthenia Gravis and Its Treatments in the Newborn

Although maternal outcomes are similar between MG patients and controls, some studies have shown that neonates from MG mothers are more likely to have lower birth weight than controls. This may be related to some medications used in pregnancy.

Newborns also have a risk of developing transient neonatal MG, which is caused by passive transfer of pathogenic antibodies through the placenta. This can be more severe when the mother has MuSK antibodies. Current estimates of the risk of neonatal MG are between 5% and 10% of live births.[2,3,6] Clinically, neonatal MG presents with hypotonia, difficulty suckling, and depressed breathing. This can be seen within hours of delivery but up to several days later; therefore, observation of the neonate for at least 2 days is recommended. Management is usually supportive, and neonates may need ventilatory support; pyridostigmine/neostigmine can be used, and rarely IVIG is needed. Symptoms are transitory and typically improve after several days; in rare cases, a fixed myopathy can leave permanent weakness.

A rare form of neonatal MG is fetal acetylcholine receptor inactivation syndrome, whereby the mother has antibodies against the fetal fragment of the acetylcholine receptor. In these cases, the mother can be asymptomatic or oligosymptomatic. The antibodies can cause severe reduction of fetal movements in utero, with multiple joint contractures leading to arthrogryposis multiplex congenita.[2] In severe cases, this can result in stillbirth. Treatment of the mother during pregnancy (even if asymptomatic) leads to reduction of circulating antibodies and can prevent the condition in subsequent pregnancies (Box 23.1).

KEY POINTS TO REMEMBER

- During pregnancy, MG symptoms worsen in approximately 30–60% of women. Exacerbations occur most often in the first trimester, final 4 weeks of gestation, and the postpartum period.
- Pyridostigmine, corticosteroids, azathioprine, and tacrolimus do not confer increased teratogenic risk and can be maintained during pregnancy. Abrupt stopping of chronic medications can lead to exacerbation and crisis and should be avoided.
- Corticosteroids, IVIG, and plasma exchange can be used to treat exacerbations during pregnancy.
- Myasthenia does not confer increased risk of obstetric complications, but follow-up in a high-risk obstetric unit is recommended.
- Intravenous magnesium should be avoided in case of preeclampsia/eclampsia. Antiepileptic medications such a levetiracetam are potential alternatives.
- Transient neonatal myasthenia can affect approximately 5–10% of newborns, and close observation for at least 2 days is recommended.

References

1. Gilhus NE, Tzartos S, Evoli A, Palace J, Burns T. Myasthenia gravis. *Nat Rev Dis Primers.* 2019;5:30.
2. Gilhus NE. Myasthenia gravis can have consequences for pregnancy and the developing child. *Front Neurol.* 2020;11:554.
3. Alharbi M, Menon D, Barnett C, Katzberg H, Sermer M, Bril V. Myasthenia gravis and pregnancy: Toronto specialty center experience. *Can J Neurol Sci.* 2021;48:767–771.
4. Banner H, Niles KM, Ryu M, Sermer M, Bril V, Murphy KE. Myasthenia gravis in pregnancy: Systematic review and case series. *Obstet Med.* 2022 Jun;15(2):108–117. doi:10.1177/1753495X211041899
5. Cahill AG, Porter TF. Immune modulating therapies in pregnancy and lactation. *Obstet Gynecol.* 2019;133:E287–E295.
6. Breiner A, Talarico R, Hawken S, Barnett C. A population-based cohort study of pregnancy outcomes in women with myasthenia gravis. *Muscle Nerve.* 2022; 65:S42.

7. Wen JC, Liu TC, Chen YH, Chen SF, Lin HC, Tsai WC. No increased risk of adverse pregnancy outcomes for women with myasthenia gravis: A nationwide population-based study. *Eur J Neurol.* 2009;16:889–894.

8. Lake AJ, Al Khabbaz A, Keeney R. Severe preeclampsia in the setting of Myasthenia Gravis. *Case Rep Obstet Gynecol.* 2017;2017:9204930. doi:10.1155/2017/9204930

24 Pregnancy in Women With Hereditary/Genetic Myopathies

Dubravka Dodig and Mark Tarnopolsky

A 26-year-old woman with limb–girdle muscular dystrophy (LGMD) type 2D presented at 18 weeks of gestation with progressive weakness and falls. Muscle strength was unchanged on examination, but she could no longer walk safely without the walker. She also had an increase in shortness of breath however, vital capacity was unchanged. Echocardiography showed new onset hypertrophic cardiomyopathy with reduced ejection fraction (35%, N >55%). She was started on furosemide and perindopril. By 35 weeks, she required a scooter, with worsening shortness of breath and spirometry reduced 1.56 L and the plan with cardiology, respirology, obstetrics, and anesthesiology consultation for a Cesarean section at 36 weeks. The child was delivered with no complications. Six months later, the patient was using a trekking pole for ambulation, lost 25 lbs., spirometry improved to 2.13 L, and the cardiac ejection fraction improved to 47% with the same medications.

What do you do now?

GENETIC MYOPATHIES AND PREGNANCY

There is limited information about the pregnancy course and birth outcomes in women with inherited myopathies, including the congenital myopathies (CMs) and the muscular dystrophies (MDs). These are a diverse group of muscle diseases primarily affecting the skeletal muscle tissue and resulting in varying degrees and distribution of weakness and/or fatigue. They are caused by mutations in different genes encoding for proteins that play important roles in muscle function and structure.

The term *myopathy* refers to either the genetic or nongenetic/acquired disorders that affect skeletal muscle causing weakness. The genetic myopathies include metabolic myopathies (e.g., mitochondrial disorders, glycogen storage disease, and fatty acid oxidation defects), CMs (e.g., central core and nemaline rod), channelopathies (e.g., periodic paralysis), and the MDs (e.g., dystrophinopathy and LGMD). Both the MDs and the CMs are caused by genetic defects that either directly (e.g., *DYS* and *SGCA*) or indirectly (e.g., *CAPN3* and *RYR1*) alter the contractile apparatus of muscle. Traditionally, the CMs were defined by distinctive histochemical or ultrastructural changes on muscle biopsy (e.g., central cores, nemaline rods, and centronuclear); however, most are now diagnosed through genetic testing (e.g., *RYR1* and *NEB*). In contrast, the MDs are diseases of muscle membrane or supporting proteins characterized by pathological evidence of ongoing muscle degeneration and regeneration and often elevated creatine kinase (CK) activity in blood.

The current review focuses on the CMs and the MDs because these are the ones that lead to fixed weakness of the limbs, trunk, and respiratory muscles and thus directly influence pregnancy. Furthermore, some of the MDs can be associated with cardiomyopathy (e.g., dystrophinopathy, sarcoglycanopathy, and titin-associated MD), and this can further complicate pregnancy.

Myotonic dystrophy type 1 (DM1) is the most common MD in adults. DM1 is a multisystem disorder of skeletal and smooth muscle transmitted by autosomal dominant inheritance. The classical form of DM1 presents in childhood, but a neonatal form also occurs. The main features of DM1 are myotonia, weakness, cataracts, dysphagia, respiratory weakness, cardiac conduction defects, and endocrinopathies.

CMs are a group of minimally progressive or nonprogressive neuromuscular conditions that are present from birth and apparent usually by early childhood. A classical type of CM is called central core disease. This condition is often confused with MD; however, the progression is usually slower and the CK is not or only minimally elevated.

There are no curative treatments for the inherited myopathies or MDs, but a multidisciplinary approach to the management of affected individuals can greatly improve quality of life and longevity.

The degree and distribution of weakness, other system involvement, and progression of disease can potentially negatively impact both pregnancy course and maternal outcomes.[7] Patients need regular obstetric monitoring to improve gestational outcomes.

Maternal Risks: Impact on Pregnancy and Delivery

Potential maternal complications include respiratory insufficiency, falls and injuries, miscarriage, ectopic pregnancies, hypertensive disease, polyhydramnios, placental abnormalities, urinary tract or respiratory infections, operative interventions, labor abnormalities, fetal presentation, and mode of delivery. Regular cardiac or pulmonary examinations are required in patients with previously known dysfunction but are also recommended at baseline prior to pregnancy in conditions at risk.

The incidence of peripartum cardiomyopathy in Duchenne/Becker muscular dystrophy (D/BMD) carriers is unknown. There are a few reports in the literature of carriers of D/BMD presenting with peripartum cardiomyopathy. Some myopathies are associated with cardiac impairments, such as cardiomyopathies (MDs and metabolic myopathies) and arrhythmia (DM1).

Concerns in the antepartum period include drug effects on the fetus and changes in the volume of distribution and glomerular filtration rate in pregnancy. Angiotensin-converting enzyme inhibitors and angiotensin receptor blockers are contraindicated due to the risk of fetopathy. Patients with stable heart failure can be started on a cardioselective β-blocker such as metoprolol. Postpartum, diuretics and β-blockers are generally safe during lactation, although propranolol, metoprolol, and carvedilol are excreted in smaller amounts compared to atenolol and sotalol.

All patients require regular monitoring for respiratory insufficiency due to the effects of the growing fetus on the diaphragm. The extent of pulmonary compromise in neuromuscular disease depends on the pattern and severity of involvement of respiratory muscles and the presence of secondary thoracic wall abnormalities (e.g., thoracic scoliosis). Maternal hypercapnia and hypoxemia can result in intrauterine death. Hence, a lung function test needs to be done in those with kyphoscoliosis and before planning pregnancy. Informing a mother to report signs of potential hypercapnia/hypoxemia such as morning headaches, nonrestorative sleep, and disordered breathing and considering nocturnal saturation studies and/or venous blood gases are recommended. The treatment of choice is noninvasive positive pressure ventilation, and maternal oxygenation should be followed with pulse oximetry.

As a general rule, women with a forced vital capacity of less than 1 L should be advised against pregnancy. In patients with significant respiratory dysfunction or rapid deterioration in pregnancy, an early delivery via cesarean section might be attempted because the beneficial effect of delivery is often immediate and dramatic.

Swallowing assessments may also be required, especially in the context of reported dysphagia to avoid poor dietary intake and maternal choking/aspiration and potential pneumonia. Dysphagia is particularly common in DM1 and nemaline rod myopathy, but it can be seen as a later manifestation in several other myopathies. A formal swallowing study and speech–language pathologist involvement are important for women report dysphagia. Most women with muscle diseases may benefit from physical and occupational therapy, given the well-known benefits of exercise for healthy maternal and offspring outcomes.

Falls pose a direct risk to the mother and a potential indirect risk to the fetus. Patients with both proximal and distal weakness are at higher fall risk, especially if there is a preexisting history of falls. Distal weakness can be seen in several MDs (e.g., DM1, facioscapulohumeral MD, and *GNE* myopathy), which can predispose to trips and falls, especially if there is superimposed proximal weakness.[3] If there is a history of tripping and/or a dorsiflexion weakness of less then 4 on 5-point MRC scale, an ankle–foot orthotic should be considered. Weakness of the hip girdle and quadriceps muscles is a risk factor for falling and functional impairments such as stair climbing or getting out of a chair. The addition of the growing fetal weight makes these activities of daily living more difficult. Patients with significant hip girdle weakness often adopt a lordotic posture and a Trendelenburg gait. Both can be worsened by the anterior displacement of the center of gravity from the growing fetus and impair the mother's ambulation. Patients often report lumbar pain and increased fatigue. The use of a cane or trekking pole can help during this period, but some patients may require a rollator walker or even a scooter if ambulation deteriorates and fall risk escalates.

Pregnant women with MD have an increased risk of preeclampsia (twofold higher than the general population), preterm premature rupture of the membranes, and preterm labor.[4] In DM, the percentage of preeclampsia is slightly increased (9%).

The high frequency of complications in pregnancy in DM1 patients is well known and includes ectopic pregnancies, placental anomalies, and urinary tract infections. It is hypothesized that the involvement of the smooth muscles plays a role in the pathogenesis. Labor may be prolonged because of muscle weakness, and there is an increased risk of instrumental delivery or cesarean section. Patients with myotonic dystrophy are also at risk of postpartum hemorrhage.

In addition to the respiratory weakness issues in some myopathies, there are several myopathies with specific anesthetic risks.[8] The best known in the increased risk of malignant hyperthermia (MH) in central core and mini-/multi-core disease due to mutations in the *RYR1* or *CACNA1S* genes. This disorder can have an untreated mortality rate of approximately 33%, with volatile inhalational anesthetics and depolarizing muscle-blocking agents being triggers. General anesthesia in affected individuals is associated with life-threatening perioperative complications, including cardiac arrhythmias, cardiac arrest, and a malignant hyperpyrexia-like syndrome.

All patients with central core and mini-/multi-core myopathy should be treated with MH precautions even in the absence of genetic testing, and any patient with a positive and permissive family history of MH should be considered as being MH positive unless proven otherwise. MH is only an issue with cesarean section, but it is more likely in myopathy patients; appropriate preventative strategies dramatically lower the risk of anesthetic complications. Although patients with other forms of MD are not at a higher risk of MH compared to the general population, there are several other concerns during anesthesia that need to be considered. First, depolarizing muscle-blocking agents can be associated with hyperkalemia. Second, the lower muscle mass requires relatively lower doses of all drugs to start with and titrate to effect (especially in DM1). Finally, the lower muscle mass also makes euthermia more difficult to maintain. All the inhalation anesthetics (desflurane, sevoflurane, isoflurane, methoxyflurane halothane, and enflurane) and succinylcholine (a depolarizing muscle relaxant) are considered to be potential MH triggers.

All patients with MD show sensitivity to medications, including opioids and sedatives and the non-depolarizing muscle relaxants.

To avoid some of the aforementioned issues, regional anesthesia is preferable to general anesthesia in patients with MDs. It avoids intubation and ventilation, which, in patients with poor lung function preoperatively, can result in significant postoperative pulmonary complications, including atelectasis. However, epidural blockade can be difficult in patients with severe spine deformities or surgically corrected scoliosis. If general anesthesia is necessary, a possible prolonged neuromuscular blockade by non-depolarizing drugs and marked sensitivity to sedative and anesthetic agents have to be considered specifically in myotonic dystrophy.

In addition to MH, mothers with central core disease can also have muscle weakness at varied levels. It is usually associated with kyphoscoliosis, osteopenia, and vitamin deficiency. The lung function can be affected in those with severe kyphoscoliosis. Other lung function abnormalities could include restrictive lung disease, respiratory muscle weakness, chest wall abnormalities, chronic aspiration, and infections leading to abnormal ventilation.

Prematurity was reported to be the major complication of DM1. Women with DM1, LGMD, and CMs are reported to be more likely to deliver by cesarean section.

Usually there is little impact on the disease course, but sometimes an impairment is noticed, which could be attributed to pregnancy and not to disease progression.[5] Awater et al.[1] reported in their case series that persistent worsening of symptoms during or after pregnancy was experienced in approximately half (54%) of LGMD pregnancies. On the contrary, temporary or lasting changes of the condition in pregnancy were not reported in DM1 or DM2, but in DM2 the first symptoms of the disease were observed in pregnancy in 6 of 42 patients (14%); walking ability was maintained in nearly all women who had been ambulant before pregnancy.

All myopathies can have a prolonged labor and delivery impact because of muscle weakness and sometimes pathologic uterine muscle. This leads to an increased risk of instrumental delivery and cesarean section. In addition, postpartum hemorrhage is not rare in DM, due to uterine atonia and abnormal position of placenta.

Neonatal Outcomes

The number of breech deliveries is highly increased for LGMD (26% of births in Awater et al.'s cohort).[1] Predictive factors of breech delivery are prematurity, low birth weight, oligohydramnios or hydramnios, and possibly also lower mother physical activity (women often in wheelchairs).

Women with LGMD and CMs are likely to deliver by cesarean section. Cesarean section is generally recommended for delivery in the presence of abnormal blood gases, vital capacity below 1–1.5 L, pulmonary hypertension or right heart failure, weak diaphragm or abdominal muscles, or pelvic abnormalities.

Fetal distress occurs frequently due to prolonged labor or affected fetuses. This is reflected by a high number of operative deliveries. Vaginal instrumentation was not increased but approximately one-third of deliveries were undertaken by cesarean section in comparison to 10–16% in a reference population.[2] The third stage of labor may be complicated by placental retention and postpartum hemorrhage.

Pregnant women with DM have a high risk of fetal loss due to early spontaneous abortion, premature delivery, or neonatal death. Second-trimester abortions are believed to be caused by functional abnormality of the uterine muscle with inability to retain the fetus.

Prematurity and poor neonatal outcome are often, but not exclusively, related to congenitally affected DM1 children. Due to the dynamic nature of the gene defect, the offspring of DM1 mothers can be severely disabled, even if the mother is only mildly affected and often unaware of her diagnosis when getting pregnant. Genetic counseling and prenatal or preimplantation genetic diagnosis are important issues in these high-risk situations. In a study on DM1, 14 of 65 newborns were congenitally affected: 2 of those died a few hours after birth and a further 3 (4.6%) were born as stillbirths.

The average Apgar score of congenitally affected children was 7.2 ± 2.2 (95% confidence interval [CI]: 6–8.4) after 10 minutes, and the score of unaffected newborns was 9.9 ± 0.4 (95% CI: 9.6–10.2).

The symptoms and signs of CMs largely depend on the type of myopathy.[6] During pregnancy, the most common symptom suggestive of an affected infant in utero is recurrent reduced fetal movements. Mothers with central core disease can have missense mutation in the *RYR1* gene, which causes muscle weakness due to sparse mitochondria and can be associated with life-threatening malignant hyperthermia. This is an autosomal dominant condition, and neonates affected by this condition may have hypotonia, muscle weakness, weak cry, and are likely to need respiratory support at birth. They usually have feeding difficulties and developmental delay. Clinical findings depend on the type of congenital myopathy and may include the following: Eyelid ptosis and extraocular muscle weakness are usually seen in multi-/mini-core disease, nemaline myopathy, and centronuclear myopathy; congenital myasthenic syndromes and respiratory insufficiency are seen in central core and multi-/mini-core diseases; cardiac involvement may be associated with multi-core disease and nemaline myopathy; dysphagia is seen with spheroid and cytoplasmic body myopathy; cognitive impairment may be seen in fingerprint myopathy and congenital fiber-type disproportion; rigid spine is associated with central core, centronuclear, multi-/mini-core, and nemaline myopathy (SELEON is the most common). Scoliosis may be an early and consistent sign.

The congenital muscular dystrophies often present in the first year with hypotonia and weakness, respiratory insufficiency, bulbar dysfunction, and arthrogryposis. Hypertrophy of the tongue and limb muscles, scoliosis, and contractures may develop with age.

Intrauterine growth restriction is reported for women with congenital dystrophy or metabolic myopathies.

Considering all of the above, clinical management of women with hereditary myopathies requires a multidisciplinary approach that includes input from an obstetrician, maternal–fetal medicine, neurologist, anesthesiologist, respirologist, cardiologist (if affected), and pediatrician/neonatologist to minimize the risk of worsening disability for the mother and/or peripartum issues for the child.

KEY POINTS TO REMEMBER

- Clinical management of women with hereditary myopathies requires a multidisciplinary approach with close follow-up and good labor planning.
- All pregnant patients require regular monitoring for cardiac and respiratory insufficiency.
- Possible complications include fetal loss; fetal growth restriction; preeclampsia and eclampsia; preterm labor; and prolonged labor and delivery, which leads to an increased risk of instrumental delivery and cesarean section.
- The perceived worsening of weakness is most commonly attributable to pregnancy and not to disease progression.

References

1. Awater C, Zerres K, Rudnik-Schöneborn S. Pregnancy course and outcome in women with hereditary neuromuscular disorders: Comparison of obstetric risks in 178 patients. *Eur J Obstet Gynecol Reprod Biol.* 2012;162(2):153–159.
2. Rudnik-Schöneborn S, Zerres K. Outcome in pregnancies complicated by myotonic dystrophy: A study of 31 patients and review of the literature. *Eur J Obstet Gynecol Reprod Biol.* 2004;114(1):44–53.
3. Ciafaloni E, Pressman EK, Loi AM, et al. Pregnancy and birth outcomes in women with facioscapulohumeral muscular dystrophy. *Neurology.* 2006; 67:1887–1889.
4. Johnson NE, Hung M, Nasser E, et al. The impact of pregnancy on myotonic dystrophy: A registry-based study. *J Neuromuscul Dis.* 2015;2(4):447–452.
5. Zagorda B, Camdessanché JP, Féasson L. Pregnancy and myopathies: Reciprocal impacts between pregnancy, delivery, and myopathies and their treatments: A clinical review. *Rev Neurol.* 2021;177(3):225–234.
6. Petrangelo A, Alshehri E, Czuzoj-Shulman N, Abenhaim HA. Obstetrical, maternal and neonatal outcomes in pregnancies affected by muscular dystrophy. *J Perinat Med.* 2018;46(7):791–796.
7. Jaffe R, Mock M, Abramowicz J, Ben-Aderet N. Myotonic dystrophy and pregnancy: A review. *Obstet Gynecol Surv.* 1986;41(5):272–278.
8. Pash MP, Balaton J, Eagle C. Anaesthetic management of a parturient with severe muscular dystrophy, lumbar lordosis and a difficult airway. *Can J Anaesth.* 1996;43(9):959–963.

25 Numbness in the Hand of a Woman During Pregnancy

Carolina Barnett-Tapia

A 36-year-old female, currently at 36 weeks of her first pregnancy, reports a painful "pins and needles" sensation in her right hand that has been worsening during the past 4 weeks. The symptoms are worse at night and awaken her; she obtains some relief by shaking the hand or changing position. During the past week, she has noted some clumsiness of her right thumb and difficulty texting on her cell phone. General exam is notable for pitting edema. Neurological examination reveals decreased sensation to pinprick in the right thumb, index finger, and third finger and minimal weakness in the abduction of the right thumb. There is no atrophy. The neurological examination is otherwise normal.

What do you do now?

CARPAL TUNNEL SYNDROME

Median neuropathy at the wrist is a very common focal neuropathy. When symptomatic, it presents as carpal tunnel syndrome (CTS), with an estimated incidence of approximately 3.4% in the general population.[1] CTS is much more prevalent in pregnant women, with prospective cohorts showing symptoms consistent with CTS in 34–60% of pregnancies, and electrophysiology confirming a median neuropathy at the wrist in up to approximately 40%.[2–5]

Anatomy and Pathophysiology

The median nerve is formed when the lateral (C6–C7) and medial cords (C8–T1) of the brachial plexus join. It gives no branches until it passes between the two heads of the pronator teres, after which it supplies the pronator teres, flexor carpi radialis, and flexor digitorum sublimus. It then gives off a pure motor branch, the anterior interosseus nerve, which supplies the flexor pollicis longus, pronator quadratus, and the medial head of the flexor digitorum profundus (supplying the second and third fingers). Right before entering the carpal tunnel, the palmar sensory branch arises, providing sensation to the thenar eminence. The median nerve then enters through the carpal tunnel proper, which is formed by carpal bones in the floor and sides and has the transverse carpal ligament for the roof. After exiting the carpal tunnel in the hand, the nerve divides into a motor branch supplying the first and second lumbricals, abductor pollicis brevis, opponens pollicis, and superficial head of flexor pollicis brevis. The sensory branch supplies the medial thumb, index and middle finger, and half of the ring finger.[1]

Given the small size of the carpal tunnel, any increase in the volume of its contents or a decrease in the size of the tunnel may lead to compression of the median nerve at this location. In pregnancy, increased fluid retention raising the pressure within the carpal tunnel likely explains the higher prevalence of median neuropathy at the wrist. Other risk factors include diabetes, hypothyroidism, rheumatoid arthritis, and trauma (e.g., Colles fracture). CTS in pregnancy usually presents in the third trimester and is more likely to be bilateral; however, it is usually milder that in the general population. Nulliparity and edema increase the likelihood of developing the disorder.[3]

Clinical Presentation

Patients with CTS present with numbness and tingling in the hand(s), which they may have difficulty localizing. Referred pain in the forearm may also occur. Symptoms are usually worse at night, and they may also be triggered by repetitive flexion and extension of the wrists. In more severe cases, patients may develop weakness in the muscles of the thumb and thenar atrophy.

Tinel sign (developing paresthesia when tapping over the median nerve at the wrist) and Phalen sign (developing paresthesia with passive wrist flexion) have low sensitivity and specificity compared to electrophysiology testing.

Examination may reveal loss of pinprick sensation in the first three digits, sometimes with splitting of the fourth finger. In more severe cases, there may be atrophy of the thenar eminence and weakness of the abductor pollicis brevis (Figure 25.1). This muscle is best tested by having

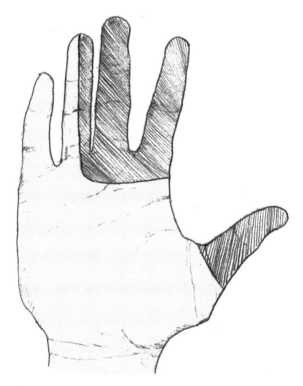

FIGURE 25.1 Sensory loss in carpal tunnel syndrome.
Illustration by J. Risien Waters.

> **BOX 25.1 Signs and Symptoms of Carpal Tunnel Syndrome**
>
> **Symptoms**
>
> - Paresthesia in one or both hands, particularly during sleep, often relieved by shaking the hand(s).
> - Pain in the forearm may occur.
> - May report dropping objects and/or clumsiness of thumb.
>
> **Possible Signs on Examination**
>
> - Reduced pinprick sensation in the palmar surface of the thumb, index finger, third digit, and median half of the fourth digit; the thenar eminence is spared.
> - Weakness of thumb abduction vertical to the plane of the palm.
> - Atrophy of the thenar eminence.

the patient place the hand in a supine position and abduct the thumb perpendicular to the plane of the palm. In CTS, interphalangic flexion of the thumb is normal because this muscle (flexor pollicis longus) is located in the forearm, proximal to the wrist, as are the branches that mediate wrist flexion, pronation, and sensation of the thenar eminence (Box 25.1).

Diagnosis

Carpal tunnel syndrome is a clinical diagnosis, whereby the typical symptoms are correlated to compression of the median nerve at the wrist. Patients with electrophysiologic findings of median neuropathy at the wrist—commonly seen in polyneuropathy—but without symptoms do not have CTS. In pregnant patients with typical and mild symptoms, electrodiagnostic testing may not be needed. However, if symptoms are severe or not responding to first-line treatment, or there are atypical features in the exam, electrodiagnostic studies are recommend. These are safe in pregnant women.

Treatment and Outcomes

Most women who develop CTS in pregnancy have a rapid resolution of symptoms after delivery. Therefore, the first line of treatment is conservative management with wrist splints at night to maintain a neutral position of the wrist(s). Avoiding repetitive wrist movements is also recommended. In patients who have limited or no response to splints, local steroid injections can provide symptomatic relief.[5] Surgical intervention is very rarely needed in pregnancy, but some women who persist with symptoms after delivery may eventually need surgery. Older studies described persistent symptoms in up to 50% of women at 12 months post-delivery; however, a large prospective cohort found this number to be much smaller, and 15% of women still had carpal tunnel symptoms 12 months after delivery.[4]

KEY POINTS TO REMEMBER

- Carpal tunnel syndrome occurs more commonly in pregnant women than in the general population.
- It usually presents in the third trimester of pregnancy and can be bilateral.
- Increased frequency is probably due to gestational fluid retention causing increased pressure with the carpal tunnel.
- First line of treatment is conservative, with wrist splints and avoidance of repetitive wrist movements. Some patients benefit form steroidal injection.
- Most patients have improvement of symptoms after delivery, but approximately 15% (one in six) will have persistent symptoms 1 year after delivery.

References

1. Preston DC, Shapiro BE. Median neuropathy at the wrist. In: *Electromyography and Neuromuscular Disorders*. 2nd ed. Elsevier; 2005;255–279.
2. Padua L, Aprile I, Caliandro P, et al. Symptoms and neurophysiological picture of carpal tunnel syndrome in pregnancy. *Clin Neurophysiol*. 2001;112:1946–1951.
3. Meems M, Truijens S, Spek V, Visser LH, Pop VJ. Prevalence, course and determinants of carpal tunnel syndrome symptoms during pregnancy: A prospective study. *BJOG*. 2015;122:1112–1118.
4. Meems M, Truijens S, Spek V, Visser LH, Pop VJ. Follow-up of pregnancy-related carpal tunnel syndrome symptoms at 12 months postpartum: A prospective study. *Eur J Obstet Gynecol Reprod Biol*. 2017;211:231–223.
5. Gooding MS, Evangelista V, Pereira L. Carpal tunnel syndrome and meralgia paresthetica in pregnancy. *Obstet Gynecol Surv*. 2020;75:121–126.

26 A Woman With Leg Weakness After Delivery

Nouf Alfaidi and Carolina Barnett-Tapia

A 32-year-old woman reported leg weakness a day after vaginal delivery. An epidural was placed on the first attempt, and labor required augmentation. After 3 hours, forceps were used to assist delivery of an 8 pound 12 ounce (3,970 g) baby. The next morning, when the patient got out of bed, she was unable to walk because her right leg buckled when standing up. She did not report back pain but noted a prickly sensation on her right upper thigh. She has had no bowel or bladder symptoms. On examination, the epidural insertion site had no firmness nor tenderness. Motor exam revealed weakness in the right iliopsoas (4/5) and quadriceps (3/5) and normal strength in all other muscles of the thigh and leg. Sensory exam revealed loss of pinprick sensation in the right anteromedial thigh. Reflex exam was notable for an absent right patellar reflex. Toes were down-going.

What do you do now?

FEMORAL NEUROPATHY

Obstetrical nerve injuries are common and occur in up to 1% of deliveries. Of these, femoral nerve injury is the most common cause of postpartum leg weakness. It occurs in approximately 2.8 per 100,000 deliveries. In 25% of patients, the injury is bilateral, causing significant impairment of mobility in new mothers.

Anatomy and Pathophysiology

The femoral nerve arises from the lumbar plexus, where nerve roots L2–L4 are joined. It passes between the iliacus and psoas muscles and then courses under the inguinal ligament.[1] During delivery, when the hip is flexed, abducted, and externally rotated in the lithotomy position, the femoral nerve may be compressed at the level of the inguinal ligament. Compression may be caused by the fetal head or by instruments in the pelvic floor. A prolonged period of time spent in the lithotomy position can increase the risk of femoral nerve injury.[2,3,4]

Clinical Presentation

Injury to the femoral nerve produces weakness in the quadriceps femoris, causing weakness of knee extension. Clinically, patients present with leg buckling upon standing because the quadriceps is unable to support the knee. If the injury occurs proximal to the inguinal ligament, there may be weakness of the iliopsoas muscle, with impairments in hip flexion, and patients may have difficulty standing from a chair. Sensory loss can occur in the anteromedial thigh, corresponding to the anterior femoral nerve, and in the medial leg, corresponding to the saphenous nerve, sensory branches of the femoral nerve (Figure 26.1). The patellar reflex is reduced or absent.

Diagnosis of femoral neuropathy can often be made at the bedside by obtaining a thorough history and clinical exam. The latter is focused on looking for any signs of involvement of other nerves or lumbosacral roots. For example, sensation of the lateral thigh should not be affected by femoral neuropathy because it is supplied by the lateral femoral cutaneous nerve derived from L2–L3. Likewise, sensation of the proximal medial thigh and thigh adduction are dependent on the obturator nerve, so they should be intact in isolated femoral neuropathy. The differential diagnosis for leg weakness

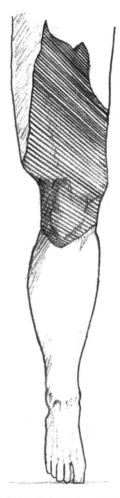

FIGURE 26.1 Sensory loss in the thigh with femoral neuropathy. This area is supplied by the intermediate and medial cutaneous nerves of the thigh, sensory branches of the femoral nerve. The saphenous branch is not depicted.

Illustration by J. Risien Waters.

in the postpartum patient is broad, and it is important to distinguish focal neuropathies (e.g., femoral) from other more ominous disorders (Box 26.1). Electrodiagnostic testing with nerve conduction studies and electromyography can help localize the lesion when the clinical presentation is atypical and can also help with prognostication in severe cases or when there is no

> **BOX 26.1 Differential Diagnosis of Postpartum Leg Weakness**
>
> - Femoral neuropathy
> - Peroneal neuropathy
> - Obturator neuropathy
> - Lumbosacral plexopathy
> - Spinal cord injury (e.g., epidural hematoma, direct spinal cord/
>   cauda equina injury, and anterior spinal artery syndrome)

significant improvement within several weeks. These studies are safe in pregnancy and postpartum, but they should be done at least 10–15 days after injury because they can be normal in the hyperacute state.

Of note, if in addition to weakness, the patient presents with pain in the back, hip, groin, and/or abdomen, with or without hemodynamic instability, this should raise the possibility of a retroperitoneal hematoma. This is a rare cause for postpartum femoral neuropathy, as the hematoma can compress the femoral nerve at the iliopsoas gutter causing leg weakness.[4] Retroperitoneal hematoma can occur postoperatively following cesarean section in the setting of bleeding diathesis or trauma. Spontaneous rupture of the uterine artery may also produce retroperitoneal hematoma. Diagnosis is made with computed tomography of the abdomen and pelvis.

Treatment and Outcome of Postpartum Femoral Neuropathy

Most femoral neuropathies during delivery are caused by focal demyelination and improve within days to several weeks. Treatment is conservative, including using a knee brace to support the leg while standing and physical therapy. In the rare case of a retroperitoneal hematoma, this might require surgical intervention.[2,3]

There is scarce evidence regarding the risk of recurrence in subsequent pregnancies and deliveries. A case report of a woman with recurrent symptoms of femoral neuropathy in a second pregnancy prompted a planned cesarean section. Given the lack of evidence, we recommend that patients with a history of pregnancy-related femoral neuropathy should have close follow-up in subsequent pregnancies.[5] In case of symptom recurrence (e.g., knee extension weakness), a multidisciplinary assessment including the obstetrics and neurology team is needed to decide whether a planned cesarean section is appropriate in a specific patient.

Other Lower Extremity Neuropathies Associated With Pregnancy and Delivery

The most common lower extremity nerve injuries associated with pregnancy and delivery in descending order of frequency are lateral femoral cutaneous nerve, femoral nerve, peroneal nerve, lumbosacral plexus, sciatic nerve, and obturator nerve. The use of epidural anesthesia in the management of labor pain may increase the risk of nerve injury due to its tendency to contribute to a prolonged second stage of labor. In addition, the absence of sensation prevents women from sensing pressure and adjusting their position. Other risk factors for obstetrical nerve injury include nulliparity, short stature, large fetus, excessive weight gain, and instrumental delivery (Box 26.2). In general, postpartum neuropathy has an excellent prognosis, with expected recovery time of 6–8 weeks.

Lateral femoral cutaneous neuropathy (meralgia paresthetica) is the most common focal neuropathy of the lower extremity during pregnancy and delivery. It is a pure sensory neuropathy and does not cause any weakness. The lateral femoral cutaneous nerve passes under the inguinal ligament where it is susceptible to compression, especially due to increased abdominal pressure such as seen in pregnancy. The nerve can also be compressed and/or stretched during delivery. Risk factors during pregnancy include large-for-gestational-age fetus, gestational diabetes, and excessive maternal weight gain. Risk factors during delivery include being nulliparous or with prolonged second stage of labor.

Lateral femoral cutaneous neuropathy presents with painful paresthesia and/or numbness in the lateral thigh. In the case of pregnancy, symptoms usually resolve in the postpartum period, and thus, only conservative

---

BOX 26.2 **Risk Factors for Obstetrical Nerve Injuries**

- Nulliparity
- Short stature
- Prolonged second stage of labor
- Instrumental delivery
- Large fetus
- Excessive weight gain
- Epidural anesthesia

management is needed. This includes avoidance of tight clothing and positions that aggravate the condition. Ultrasound-guided corticoid injections can be used in cases of severe pain, but this is rarely needed in pregnancy.

Injuries to the lumbosacral plexus can occur during delivery due to compression from the fetal head or forceps at the pelvic brim. Symptoms are dependent on the nerve roots involved, most commonly the L4 and L5 nerve roots, causing weakness in ankle dorsiflexion, inversion, and eversion. Sensory impairment is predominantly in the distribution of the L5 dermatome. Risk factors include large fetal size, small maternal size, fetal malposition, and instrumental delivery.

Fibular (peroneal) neuropathy is usually caused by compression of the peroneal nerve at the fibular head. In the obstetrical population, it has been attributed to prolonged knee flexion while squatting, lithotomy position, or pressure on the fibular head during delivery. Patients present with weakness in foot dorsiflexion causing foot drop, weakness of first toe extension, and foot eversion. Patients may report decreased sensation of pinprick on the dorsum of the foot, most pronounced between the first and second toes. Awareness of the vulnerability to nerve injuries during obstetrical procedures has led to appropriate repositioning and decreased frequency of injury.

Obturator neuropathy is rare and represents less than 5% of all postpartum neuropathies. Patients present with weakness of thigh adduction and sensory loss of the upper third of the medial thigh. Patients with this disorder will have a wide-based gait with circumduction. Risk factors include large fetal head and instrumental vaginal delivery. Management is conservative, with emphasis on physical therapy.

Other Causes of Postpartum Leg Weakness

An epidural hematoma is an extremely rare but serious cause of postpartum leg weakness. It occurs in 1 in 200,000 patients after spinal anesthesia and in 1 in 150,000 patients after epidural anesthesia.[6] Acute interscapular pain during labor may indicate the formation of a spinal epidural hematoma. Patients usually present with back pain, interscapular pain and tenderness, persistent anesthesia, numbness, weakness, and sphincter dysfunction. Risk factors include use of antiplatelet agents and anticoagulants, inherited or acquired clotting dysfunction, low platelet count, and the presence of spine and nerve root tumors (Box 26.3). The diagnosis is confirmed with magnetic resonance imaging (MRI) of the spine, and urgent neurosurgical consultation is required.

Anterior spinal artery syndrome is an extremely rare entity in the setting of epidural anesthesia. Potential risks factors include intraoperative hypotension, toxicity from local anesthesia, or vasospasm related to the administration of a local epinephrine-containing anesthetic. Other causes of spinal cord infarction include atherosclerosis of the aorta, aortic dissection or aortic surgery, spinal arteriovenous malformations, postpartum hypercoagulopathy, and air embolism.[7]

Patients with anterior spinal artery ischemia present with acute paraplegia, loss of pain and temperature sensation, and bowel and bladder dysfunction. Proprioception and vibration perception are spared. The presence of bowel and bladder dysfunction and the diffuse weakness and sensory loss distinguish this injury from bilateral neuropathies. Spine MRI is essential to exclude other causes and to confirm the diagnosis of cord infarction.

Injury to the conus medullaris during administration of neuraxial block is extremely rare. It occurs if there is inadvertent placement of the catheter at a higher level than L2. Patients may experience leg weakness, pain, saddle anesthesia, and bowel and bladder dysfunction.

KEY POINTS TO REMEMBER

- Femoral neuropathy is the most common cause of postpartum leg weakness after delivery.

> BOX 26.3 **Predisposing Factors for Epidural Hematoma**
>
> - Gestational thrombocytopenia
> - Preeclampsia/eclampsia/HELLP (hemolytic anemia, elevated liver enzymes, and low platelets) syndrome
> - Inherited clotting dysfunction
> - Acquired clotting dysfunction
> - Spinal cord and nerve root tumor

- Hallmarks of femoral neuropathy include leg buckling due to weakness in knee extensors, numbness and paresthesia in the anteromedial thigh and medial leg, and reduced or absent patellar reflex.
- Postpartum neuropathy generally has an excellent prognosis. Treatment is conservative in most cases, and patients usually have significant improvement within 6–8 weeks.
- Complications of epidural anesthetic and retroperitoneal hematoma are very rare causes of leg weakness after delivery, but they should be suspected in cases of sphincter dysfunction, saddle anesthesia, or severe back or groin pain.

References

1. Preston DC, Shapiro BE. Femoral neuropathy. In: *Electromyography and Neuromuscular Disorders*. 2nd ed. Elsevier; 2005:355–364.
2. O'Neal A, Chang L, Salajeghi K. Postpartum spinal cord, root, plexus and peripheral nerve injuries involving lower extremities: A practical approach. *Anesth Analg*. 2014;120(1):141–148.
3. O'Neal MA. Lower extremity weakness and numbness in the postpartum period: A case-based review. *Neurol Clin*. 2019;37(1):103–111. doi:10.1016/j.ncl.2018.09.002
4. Chao A, Chao A, Wang CJ, Chao AS. Femoral neuropathy: A rare complication of retroperitoneal hematoma caused by cesarean section. *Arch Gynecol Obstet*. 2013;287(3):609–611. doi:10.1007/s00404-012-2527-8
5. Chow K, Wong K, Gill A. Severe postpartum femoral neuropathy: A case series. *J Obstet Gynaecol Can*. 2021;43(5):603–606. doi:10.1016/j.jogc.2020.07.015
6. Hsu JL, Chin SC, Cheng MH, Wu YR, Ro A, Ro LS. Postpartum spinal cord infarction: A case report and review of the literature. *Medicines*. 2022;9(11):54. doi:10.3390/medicines9110054
7. Raasck K, Habis AA, Aoude A, et al. Spontaneous spinal epidural hematoma management: A case series and literature review. *Spinal Cord Ser Cases*. 2017;3:16043. doi:10.1038/scsandc.2016.43

SECTION VI

Neuro-Infectious Disease

27 "I Can't Concentrate at Work"

Caleb R. S. McEntire, George K. Harrold, and Kathleen Miller

A 58-year-old woman who works as a paralegal is referred to your outpatient clinic for difficulties with concentration. Her medical history is significant HIV diagnosed 19 years ago. She had a $CD4^+$ T-cell count of 98 cells/µl on first presenting to medical care, she has since been strictly adherent to her antiretroviral therapy (ART) regimen of tenofovir alafenamide, emtricitabine, and bictegravir with normal $CD4^+$ T-cell count and undetectable serum viral load for many years. She reports difficulty with memory, concentration, and decision-making. She scores 28/30 on the Montreal Cognitive Assessment. On the HIV Dementia Scale she scores 10/12. MRI shows mild but diffuse subcortical white matter abnormalities, and a lumbar puncture does not show detectable HIV virus. She is referred for cognitive therapy and maintained on her current ART.

What do you do now?

HIV ENCEPHALOPATHY AND DEMENTIA

People living with HIV can experience cognitive impairments that affect their memory, concentration, attention, and motor skills. When cognitive impairments are not clearly attributable to another cause besides HIV infection, they are collectively known as HIV-associated neurocognitive disorders (HAND). These issues can occur and progress even when patients are appropriately treated with good virologic control. Even in the post-ART era, neurocognitive impairment, ranging from asymptomatic cognitive impairment to more severe deficits, can occur in up to one-third of people with HIV (PWH). Low nadir CD4+ T-cell count correlates with severity of cognitive dysfunction in HAND even if counts have subsequently been well controlled, possibly because of HIV reservoirs that can remain in the central nervous system (CNS) after initial viral infiltration across the blood–brain barrier. Women with HAND may have more severe disease likely due to a variety of socioeconomic factors, including higher barriers to education and health care at baseline. Specific MRI modalities, in addition to standard volumetric MRI, may help diagnose or track HAND. Initiation of effective ART is the most important element in treatment of the condition, although HAND may persist even with appropriate ART.

The Changing Epidemiology of HIV

In the United States, an estimated 1.2 million people were living with HIV at the end of 2019, a prevalence of approximately 0.3% of adults. Men who have sex with men remain the group with the highest incidence, but Black and Hispanic people are now disproportionately affected by HIV with a recent rise in cases. Incidence of HIV has increased among both cisgender and transgender women in recent years. In particular, transgender women are at very high risk of acquiring HIV, with 40% of transgender women recently surveyed in the United States identifying as having HIV. In addition, the proportion of new infections occurring among cisgender women has more than doubled from 1981 to 2019, from 8% to 18%. These numbers also vary globally; in sub-Saharan Africa, 60% of PWH are women, and in Latin America, Eastern Europe, Central Asia, and East Asia, 30–35% of PWH are women.[1]

Although men comprise the majority of PWH worldwide, studies on HIV and cognition have nevertheless disproportionately underrepresented women. In a review of neuropsychological complications of HIV, only 31% of 236 studies from 1988 to 1997 included women with representation proportional to their prevalence in the population.[2]

The prevalence of HIV-related neurocognitive changes in women compared to men has been estimated variously as equivalent, slightly higher, or up to twice as high.[3] This may represent a variety of socioeconomic and psychosocial challenges that women at risk for HIV infection face—including high rates of poverty, lower access to formal education, and barriers to health care access—rather than representing an intrinsic host or disease factor. However, the rates of depression among women living with HIV are significantly higher than those among men, and so a contribution of pseudodementia or psychiatric illness could also have an effect.

HIV Dementia: Classification and Presentation

HIV-associated neurocognitive disorder comprises a spectrum of neurologic and psychological impairments that can occur and progress in PWH even with good viral control. The most recent American Academy of Neurology nomenclature classifies HAND into three categories of ascending severity: asymptomatic neurocognitive impairment (ANI), mild neurocognitive disorder (MND), and HIV-associated dementia (HAD).[4]

MND often presents with cognitive deficits that affect attention, working memory, executive functioning, and speed of information processing. Although most HIV-positive patients with such cognitive impairments display no evident symptoms or impairment in functioning (ANI), some may develop subtle symptoms such as difficulty with complex tasks, maintaining concentration, or reading. Unlike the subacute onset of classic HAD, cognitive deficits in milder forms of HAND have a more chronic onset and can remain stable or progress very slowly over years.

Motor problems are not common in milder cases of HAND, but if present, they can include unsteady gait, slowed fine hand coordination, and tremors. Affective disturbances, such as apathy, lethargy, loss of sexual drive, and diminished emotional responsiveness, can also be associated with HAND. Brain imaging and routine cerebrospinal fluid (CSF) studies are not effective at distinguishing between patients with HIV without neurocognitive impairment and those with mild neurocognitive deficits. Although cerebral atrophy or white matter abnormalities may be observed in some patients, imaging is often normal in patients with milder forms of HAND.

The classic form of HAD is chiefly distinguished by subcortical dysfunction that manifests in attention and concentration deficits, depressive symptoms, and impaired psychomotor speed and accuracy. This and the lack of cortical syndromes, such as aphasias or agnosias, align with research indicating that HIV primarily impacts subcortical and deep gray matter structures. HAD is more prevalent among patients with untreated, advanced HIV infection, and its onset typically occurs in a subacute manner. Unlike with primary neurodegenerative disorders, HAD can fluctuate over time, consistent with its inflammatory-mediated etiology.[5]

Pathogenesis, Epidemiology, and Predictors of HAND

Cognitive deficits can occur and progress in PWH, even in patients who are virologically suppressed. The pathogenesis of this is still incompletely understood, but it may involve chronic neuroinflammation mediated at least in part by CNS compartmentalization of HIV-specific antibodies that are functionally unaffected by ART.

Since the introduction of ART, the prevalence of severe cognitive sequelae of HIV/AIDS has decreased dramatically. The CASCADE cohort (Concerted Action on Seroconversion to AIDS and Death in Europe) followed 15,380 PWH longitudinally and demonstrated a nearly 10-fold reduction in the incidence of HAD, the most severe manifestation of HAND, from pre-ART to post-ART eras (6.49 per 1,000 person-years to 0.66 per 1,000 person-years).[6] By contrast, the prevalence of milder forms of HAND in the post-ART era is similar to that in the pre-ART era, or perhaps even higher; up to half of PWH who have well-controlled disease on ART may have subclinical or mild cognitive changes. Prevalence estimates for specific HAND diagnoses in a cohort study of 1,555 PWH within the United States from 2003 to 2007 included 33% of patients with ANI, 12% with mild MNI, and 2% with HAD. The strongest predictor of impairment was history of a low CD4+ T-cell nadir, even if this measure had subsequently increased on therapy.[7]

Sex Differences in HAND

Although a number of studies have examined cognition in women with HIV, the Women's Interagency HIV Study is the largest longitudinal cohort to do so, and it represents a demographically similar cohort to the population of women living with HIV in the United States.[8] The only cognitive deficits in this study that could clearly be attributed to HIV infection were small effects in the domains of verbal learning and memory, speed of information processing, and attention. However, baseline characteristics such as reading level, age, years of education, and race were more strongly associated with performance compared to HIV status. Risk factors associated with greater deficits in patients with HIV were fewer years of education, low $CD4^+$ T-cell nadir, high viral load, and history of an AIDS-defining illness.

Only a limited number of studies have directly compared the neurocognitive performance of men and women living with HIV. These studies were limited by low sample size and confounding factors, but some showed trends toward very slightly higher rates of cognitive impairment in women compared to men with HIV (55% vs. 52%)[9] and more severe impairment in verbal memory for texts specifically (42% vs. 10%). Other studies have not found sex to be a significant predictor of cognitive impairment in PWH.

Diagnosis of HAND

New or progressive cognitive deficits may indicate the presence of HAND in PWH. However, accurate diagnosis of HAND requires ruling out other disorders that could contribute to cognitive impairment, including neurodegenerative or neurologic conditions, psychiatric disorders, substance use disorders, and medication side effects. This process of excluding alternate conditions must be determined on an individual basis and could include serologic testing, imaging, or CSF analysis. Focal or cortical symptoms should raise suspicion for a pathology other than HAND. In addition, comorbid conditions should be carefully managed. Clinical assessment can be performed with reasonable accuracy using the HIV Dementia Scale,[10] which provides a relatively sensitive and specific measure of the subcortical deficits often seen in HAND.

MRI offers a variety of methods to assess HIV-related changes in the brain. Standard volumetric MRI can show cortical and subcortical volume loss even in patients receiving adequate treatment for the disease, and the proportion of volume loss appears to correlate with degree of cognitive impairment at least in more advanced stages of disease and likely in earlier stages of disease. MR spectroscopy (MRS) may offer a more sensitive modality because it appears to correlate with degree of CNS inflammation and neuronal injury in the context of HIV infection, although it can have a latency of 6–12 months to correlate with cognitive symptoms. MRS changes are best measured in frontal white matter and basal ganglia, and glutamatergic compounds (glutamate and glutamine) appear to offer the most sensitive measure of HIV-mediated neuroinflammation. Diffusion tensor imaging may also offer a useful marker of HAND, showing lower fractional anisotropy and higher mean diffusivity in PWH than in healthy control groups primarily in the corpus callosum, although this is still in early stages of characterization.

HAND Prognosis and Response to Treatment

Antiretroviral therapy remains the mainstay of treatment for HAND. Data show a significant improvement in neurocognitive performance in patients with HAD once on ART. There has been a significant decrease in the incidence of HAD in the era of ART. In contrast, the impact of ART on milder forms of HAND is less clear.

Although there is no clear best choice of ART for management of HAND, initiation of ART in PWH is clearly associated with a better cognitive prognosis. Early initiation of therapy in PWH who have significant CD4+ lymphopenia leads to better outcomes, whereas early versus late initiation of therapy may be approximately equivalent in those with relatively preserved proxies of immune function. Women with cognitive deficits due to HAND do appear to respond to treatment, at least in the early stages of disease. One study of 126 women with HAND showed neurocognitive performance among patients receiving HAART improved significantly between baseline testing and an 18-month follow-up, whereas an untreated control group showed declining performance.[4]

Some current approaches focus largely on CSF-specific effects of specific ARTs. The CNS Penetration Effectiveness score is a system used to rank the efficacy of drugs in penetrating the CNS and treating HIV infection in the brain, although its utility is controversial due to its categorical scoring, lack of weighting for different criteria, and lack of consideration for toxic effects or drug interactions; it is rarely used in actual clinical practice.

Maraviroc, a CCR5 receptor antagonist, was initially identified as a potential target for highly active antiretroviral therapy (HAART) intensification due to its CNS penetrance and inhibition of viral replication in monocyte/macrophage cells. A recent pilot study involving PWH with viral suppression and stable ART for 12 months found that maraviroc-intensified HAART improved global neurocognitive performance at both 6 and 12 months without significant side effects,[11] suggesting that this could be an option in patients with HAND, although data are limited.

By contrast, efavirenz may be a more neurotoxic agent that should be avoided in PWH at risk for HAND. Its major metabolite, 8-hydroxy-efavirenz, is neurotoxic in vitro, and the medication has primarily neurocognitive adverse effects, including impaired concentration, anxiety, sleep disturbance, and depression. Symptoms usually peak within approximately 1 week of taking the medication and largely self-resolve within approximately 1 month, but some studies have shown mild neurocognitive effects persisting for years in some patients. It has also been associated with cognitive disorders in PWH who have otherwise well-controlled disease. As such, it is our recommendation to avoid efavirenz when possible in PWH with signs of cognitive impairment.

Outside of specific HAART regimens, management of comorbidities appears to play a prominent role in cognitive decline in PWH. The recent CHARTER study found that chronic illnesses including diabetes, hypertension, neuropathic pain, chronic pulmonary disease, overall frailty, and depression predicted neurocognitive decline, as did lifetime cannabis use. In this study, HIV disease and treatment characteristics were not predictive of neurocognitive decline, raising the question of how much HIV is intrinsically responsible for HAND. Regardless of this latter point, effective management of chronic disease as part of a multidisciplinary care team should be a key part of management with any PWH.

Overall, although there are not clear data on how to manage HAND outside of ART and virologic suppression, it is a common problem among both men and women with HIV. It is crucial to ensure that there are no other treatable comorbid conditions leading to cognitive decline and to provide ongoing support to patients with HAND.

KEY POINTS TO REMEMBER

- Neurocognitive impairment disorders (collectively known as HAND) are relatively common among PWH, and they are potentially more common among women living with HIV than men.
- Diagnosis of HAND is clinical based on exclusion of other causes of neurocognitive decline in PWH, although changes can sometimes be seen on MRI.
- Treatment involves ART with good virologic control and supportive care.
- Management of comorbidities of HIV may be as important as, or more important than, control of HIV itself in terms of minimizing cognitive decline.

References

1. Joint United Nations Programme on HIV/AIDS. *2008 report on the global AIDS epidemic.* World Health Organization; 2008.
2. Fox-Tierney RA, Ickovics JR, Cerreta CL, Ethier KA. Potential sex differences remain understudied: A case study of the inclusion of women in HIV/AIDS-related neuropsychological research. *Rev Gen Psychol.* 1999;3(1):44–54.
3. Robertson KR, Kapoor C, Robertson WT, Fiscus S, Ford S, Hall CD. No gender differences in the progression of nervous system disease in HIV infection. *JAIDS J Acquir Immune Defic Syndr.* 2004;36(3):817–822.
4. Cohen RA, Boland R, Paul R, Tashima K, Schoenbaum DD, Schuman DK, et al. AIDS. 2001;15:341–345. doi: 10.1097/00002030-200102160-00007.
5. McArthur JC, Haughey N, Gartner S, et al. Human immunodeficiency virus–associated dementia: An evolving disease. *J Neurovirol.* 2003;9(2):205–221.
6. Bhaskaran K, Mussini C, Antinori A, et al. Changes in the incidence and predictors of human immunodeficiency virus–associated dementia in the era of highly active antiretroviral therapy. *Ann Neurol.* 2008;63(2):213–221.
7. Heaton R, Clifford D, Franklin D, et al. HIV-associated neurocognitive disorders persist in the era of potent antiretroviral therapy: CHARTER study. *Neurology.* 2010;75(23):2087–2096.
8. Maki PM, Rubin LH, Valcour V, et al. Cognitive function in women with HIV: Findings from the Women's Interagency HIV Study. *Neurology.* 2015;84(3):231–240.
9. Faílde-Garrido JM, Alvarez MR, Simón-López MA. Neuropsychological impairment and gender differences in HIV-1 infection. *Psychiatry Clin Neurosci.* 2008;62(5):494–502.

10. Power C, Selnes OA, Grim JA, McArthur JC. HIV Dementia Scale: A rapid screening test. *JAIDS J Acquir Immune Defic Syndr.* 1995;8(3):273–278.

11. Gates TM, Cysique LA, Siefried KJ, et al. Maraviroc-intensified combined antiretroviral therapy improves cognition in virally suppressed HIV-associated neurocognitive disorder. *AIDS.* 2016;30(4):591–600. 10.1097/QAD.0000000000000951

28 A Woman With Headache and Confusion

Caleb R. S. McEntire and
Miriam B. Barshak

An 84-year-old woman presents to an emergency room for evaluation of headache and confusion. She is oriented to "a hospital" but thinks the year is 2001. Her daughter confirms that she was at her "very sharp" baseline a week ago. Confidentially, the patient reveals to you that she had an isolated, painless genital lesion about a year ago that resolved spontaneously. On physical examination, her neck is stiff to passive movement. She has fever to 102.6°F. MRI reveals a small stroke in the right middle cerebral artery territory. RPR is positive at 1:32 and FTA-ABS is reactive. Lumbar puncture shows 306 nucleated cells with 96% lymphocytes/μl and protein 133 mg/dl, as well as positive CSF VDRL test at titer of 1:8. She is admitted and receives aqueous crystalline penicillin G at a dose of 3 million units intravenously every 4 hours for 10 days, and she recovers well.

What do you do now?

NEUROSYPHILIS

Syphilis is a blood- and body fluid–transmitted infection caused by the bacterium *Treponema pallidum pallidum* that can affect nearly any organ system. Although historically considered a disease predominantly affecting men, the rate of syphilis has been rising in women, as well as older patients, during the past two decades. The rates of intrapartum syphilis and associated congenital syphilis infections have also risen both in the United States and globally. Neurosyphilis is a relatively common complication of systemic syphilis, and although some manifestations of neurosyphilis are often framed as occurring only in association with specific stages of systemic syphilis, any neurosyphilis phenotype can occur during essentially any stage of systemic disease. Treatment with appropriate penicillin formulations is generally very effective in halting disease course and often in reversing effect, although in late neurosyphilis with parenchymal disease, there is rarely complete recovery. Treatment of birthing parents during pregnancy is highly effective in reducing both intrapartum complications and rates of vertical disease transmission. Appropriate monitoring of neurosyphilis after treatment includes clinical monitoring and serial examinations of serum and CSF.

Clinical Presentation

Syphilis is an infection caused by the spirochete *Treponema pallidum pallidum*. Transmitted by blood and body fluids, the initial stage of disease, primary syphilis, is characterized by an isolated, painless chancre at the site of inoculation, usually on the genitals, anus, or mouth. If left untreated, primary syphilis can progress to secondary syphilis, typically occurring approximately 4–10 weeks after initial chancre appearance. Secondary syphilis is characterized by a wide range of symptoms from protean, such as fever, fatigue, and generalized adenopathy, to more specific, such as a rash that may involve the palms and soles, condyloma latum, patchy alopecia, periostitis, and hepatitis. In the absence of treatment, the signs and symptoms of secondary syphilis often resolve within 2–6 weeks, at which point patients enter the latent phase of disease. In the early latent phase (approximately 1 year from symptom onset), symptoms can recur in approximately 20–25% of patients, whereas relapses in the late latent phase are uncommon.

Tertiary syphilis indicates involvement of the cardiovascular system or gummatous disease.

Treponema pallidum can invade the nervous system within days of initial symptomatic infection, and from there it can cause symptomatic or asymptomatic disease. Neurosyphilis can be divided into early and late manifestations. Although early neurosyphilis is often associated with secondary syphilis and late neurosyphilis with the tertiary stage, neurosyphilis can occur during any stage of systemic syphilis infection with or without systemic stigmata of disease. Early manifestations generally affect the vasculature, meninges, or sensory organs, whereas late forms affect the parenchyma of the brain and spinal cord.

The most common phenotypes of early neurosyphilis are asymptomatic infection, meningitis, and meningovascular disease. Sensory organ disease in the form of otosyphilis or ocular syphilis is technically a distinct disease but is often grouped with neurosyphilis. Asymptomatic neurologic involvement of *T. pallidum* appears quite common; up to 40% of patients with primary, secondary, or early latent syphilis who lack neurologic symptoms have CSF pleocytosis, and up to 30% have reactive CSF VDRL testing.[1] Current recommendations do not endorse screening for asymptomatic neurosyphilis with lumbar puncture (LP) or other invasive testing. Symptomatic meningitis most often presents within approximately 1 year of secondary infection, although it can present years or even decades later. It manifests with classic signs of fever, headache, confusion, and nuchal rigidity, and it generally presents with inflammatory CSF with lymphocytic pleocytosis in the range of 200–400 cells/µl. Cranial nerve involvement can be present, most often affecting nerves II, VII, or VIII. Unlike meningitis from other causes, MRI can rarely have specific findings of meningeal enhancement, cranial nerve enhancement, and intracranial or extramedullary spinal gummas. Gummas are more common in men but are overall uncommon in the disease; however, they can lead to a rapid diagnosis of neurosyphilis if found.

Meningovascular syphilis is variably grouped under early or late manifestations of neurosyphilis. Its prevalence peaks approximately 7 years after primary syphilis symptoms, but it can occur at any time and is often preceded by a prodrome of syphilitic meningitis symptoms. It most characteristically presents with strokes in the middle cerebral artery territory, but it can present with strokes or silent infarcts in essentially any vascular territory, including both anterior and posterior circulation. MRA has been documented to show both intracranial and extracranial vascular abnormalities, including vessel caliber irregularity and concentric vessel wall enhancement, in many cases presenting with large arterial territory strokes. However, no data exist to describe the precise sensitivity or specificity of this imaging modality.

Late forms of neurosyphilis include so-called general paresis and tabes dorsalis. General paresis refers to a progressive dementing illness that most often occurs decades after primary syphilis infection, although in rare cases it can occur as little as 2 years afterwards. Although general paresis accounted for approximately 10% of all psychiatric hospital admissions in the first half of the 20th century, it is now relatively rare given improvements in diagnosing and treating syphilis. General paresis can present with broad neuropsychological manifestations, including cognitive and memory impairments, emotional lability, and psychotic symptoms such as paranoia and delusional thinking. Tabes dorsalis classically presents with profoundly impaired proprioception, a sensory gait ataxia, hyporeflexia, bowel and bladder dysfunction, and excruciating lancinating pain crises in the abdomen.

Ocular syphilis and otosyphilis are distinct from neurosyphilis but can similarly occur during any stage of infection. Neither sensory organ manifestation carries particularly distinct features that can be used to diagnose the disease on the basis of ophthalmologic or otologic exam. Diagnosis must be made with serum testing and inspection for other systemic syphilis.

Ocular syphilis most commonly causes posterior uveitis or panuveitis but can affect any part of the eye. It can occur during any stage of syphilis and can occur either in isolation or in the context of neurosyphilis. Recent Centers for Disease Control and Prevention (CDC) guidelines recommend LP if ocular symptoms occur in conjunction with focal neurologic abnormalities. If ocular symptoms occur with reactive syphilis serology and an abnormal ophthalmologic examination but no neurologic signs or symptoms, CSF examination is not necessary.[2] Otosyphilis is less commonly diagnosed than ocular syphilis, although it may be underdiagnosed. It generally presents with hearing loss, tinnitus, or both, and systemic syphilis symptoms often accompany it. Recommendations for CSF examination in otosyphilis mirror those in ocular syphilis; LP is indicated if focal neurologic abnormalities are present.[2]

Diagnosis

Serologic and spinal fluid testing for syphilis can be divided into the broad categories of nontreponemal and treponemal testing. Nontreponemal tests are an indirect method of testing that detect the presence of cardiolipin-reactive biomarkers that are released in the course of treponeme-induced tissue damage. These include the commonly used RPR and VDRL tests. They are semiquantitative, generally being reported as an antibody titer based on quantity of IgM and IgG present, and are relatively nonspecific due to the indirect nature of their testing. Treponemal tests are based on the detection of treponemal antigens and include FTA-ABS and *T. pallidum* enzyme immunoassay. Although they were traditionally significantly more expensive than nontreponemal tests and so were used as confirmatory testing if nontreponemal screening returned positive, in recent years they have become relatively affordable and so are used increasingly as first-line tests. Nontreponemal tests often wane in titer over time after initial infection regardless of treatment status, whereas treponemal tests nearly always remain positive lifelong.

Diagnosis of suspected neurosyphilis should begin with serum treponemal and nontreponemal testing. If both tests are reactive, this indicates recent syphilis infection and can be consistent with early neurosyphilis. Reactive treponemal testing with nonreactive nontreponemal testing is consistent with either treated or more distant untreated infection, and it can be seen in patients with later manifestations of neurosyphilis. Nonreactive treponemal testing nearly always indicates no prior syphilis infection, and so further testing is not indicated unless there is a positive nontreponemal test, in which case a second treponemal test of a different type should be performed to determine whether the nontreponemal test is falsely positive. If the patient's clinical presentation and serologies are both consistent with neurosyphilis, LP should be performed with the standard cell counts and chemistries, as well as CSF VDRL. Of note, recent studies indicate a high specificity but relatively modest sensitivity of CSF VDRL of approximately 70%, so lymphocytic pleocytosis in the correct clinical context can be considered diagnostic of the disease even if CSF VDRL is negative. CSF FTA-ABS is less specific than CSF VDRL but more sensitive; this test may be helpful in cases with negative CSF VDRL testing despite strong clinical suspicion for neurosyphilis. Analysis of CSF is not indicated in patients without neurologic signs or symptoms, which can include acute or chronic altered mentation in addition to more focal neurologic deficits.[3] All patients with syphilis should be screened for additional sexually transmitted infections, including HIV.

Changing Epidemiology of Syphilis

Syphilis was historically most common in younger men (often in the third through fifth decades of life) who were sexually active or who engaged in intravenous drug use. During the past decade, however, its prevalence has been increasing globally in geriatric populations as well as in women.[4] Although rates of primary and secondary syphilis infection are lower among women than men, rates have increased substantially in the past decade. From 2014 to 2018, the prevalence of primary and secondary syphilis doubled among women, and from 2017 to 2021, it increased by 217.4%.[5] Of note, the prevalence of syphilis cases among pregnant individuals increased broadly between 2012 and 2016 across all races, ages, and ethnicities, and the rates of congenital syphilis increased 27.5% among live births. The global prevalence of syphilis in pregnant individuals in 2016 was 0.69% (473 per 100,000 live births).[6]

Individuals can be considered at high risk for infection with syphilis if they have a history of sexually transmitted infection (STI) during pregnancy, a history of drug abuse or misuse, have sex with multiple partners without barrier protection, enter prenatal care in the second trimester or later, or have a partner with a known STI. A recent study in Brazil examining risk factors in women specifically found that the strongest predictors of syphilis during pregnancy were having only one to three prenatal appointments and a previous history of STI, although other factors included incomplete basic education, four or more pregnancies, three or more sexual partners in the year preceding pregnancy, and use of illicit drugs by either the pregnant individual or their partner. However, universal screening for syphilis in pregnancy is critical because only approximately half of pregnant patients with syphilis have a discretely identifiable risk factor.[7]

Intrapartum Syphilis: Diagnosis and Treatment

Syphilis presents in pregnancy as it does outside of pregnancy, and so clinical examination during symptomatic phases can reveal the diagnosis. The birthing complications of syphilis can include preterm labor, stillbirth, and neonatal death. Vertical transmission can occur during both early and late latent stages of the disease. The risk of vertical transmission of syphilis varies with degree of birthing parent spirochetemia and stage of disease, with primary and secondary syphilis conferring the highest rates of adverse outcomes. In general, however, rates of transmission are relatively high; up to 60% of infants birthed by a parent with untreated syphilis are diagnosed with congenital syphilis. The clinical spectrum of congenital syphilis in live births can include early manifestations of hepatosplenomegaly, osteochondritis, "snuffles" (syphilitic rhinitis), iritis, and a potentially desquamatory rash. If untreated, disease can progress to bony and dental deformities, interstitial keratitis, sensorineural hearing loss, and intellectual disability, among other sequelae.

According to CDC guidelines, all pregnant individuals should be screened for syphilis at their first prenatal visit using both treponemal and nontreponemal testing. Patients at high risk for STIs should receive an additional screening at 28–32 weeks gestational age. The order of these tests is not crucial, and they can be done in accordance with individual hospital and lab testing protocols. However, false positives within both categories of tests are very common in pregnant individuals, with estimated false-positive rates of up to 83%. As such, patients with positive initial results should receive subsequent confirmatory testing. Any patients with convincingly positive results should receive treatment with intravenous penicillin G benzathine, which is effective in treatment of maternal and fetal infection. Patients who have a listed penicillin allergy should be evaluated to ensure that this is a true allergy and desensitized if so. Effective treatment of syphilis in the birthing parent can reduce stillbirths and neonatal deaths by approximately 80%.

Follow-Up After Treatment of Neurosyphilis

Patients with early neurosyphilis manifestations who receive appropriate treatment for neurosyphilis often show substantial improvement in symptoms, whereas those with late neurosyphilis generally stop progressing symptomatically and may have more limited clinical improvement, likely because the intraparenchymal effect of late manifestations can cause some degree of irreversible damage. A single-center retrospective study followed the course of 29 patients with treated neurosyphilis without HIV and found that 8 (27.6%) fully recovered, 16 (55.2%) partially recovered, and 5 (17.2%) had no improvement at all. The study noted 3 cases of treatment failure characterized by worsening symptoms and CSF parameters. Among patients with early neurosyphilis, 42% recovered completely, whereas of patients with late neurosyphilis, none recovered completely and 33% had no post-treatment recovery.[8]

Cure of systemic syphilis is defined as a fourfold decline in initial serum nontreponemal titers 12 months after the time of treatment for primary, secondary, or early latent syphilis; or 24 months after treatment for late latent or tertiary syphilis or disease of unknown duration.[3] Up to 44% of patients with syphilis may have a so-called serofast state after effective treatment in which titers never become nonreactive. Treponemal testing remains positive despite treatment and therefore is not used to monitor the status of infection following treatment. For patients with neurosyphilis, after acute treatment and recovery, CDC guidelines previously recommended serial CSF evaluations at 6-month intervals until pleocytosis resolves but more recently support use of the serum RPR titer alone, without serial CSF examinations, for people who lack HIV infection or for people with HIV infection who are on antiretroviral therapy and have serologic and clinical responses after neurosyphilis treatment.[3]

> **KEY POINTS TO REMEMBER**
>
> - The prevalence of syphilis in women, including women in the geriatric population and pregnant women, has been increasing steadily during the past decade.
> - Lumbar puncture is indicated in people suspected to have neurosyphilis based on positive serologic tests and neurologic signs or symptoms. Patients with no neurologic signs or symptoms, even those with ocular syphilis or otosyphilis, do not require CSF analysis.

- All patients with syphilis should be screened for additional sexually transmitted infections, including HIV.
- Cure of neurosyphilis can be inferred from normalization of the serum RPR titer for patients without HIV infection or patients with HIV infection who are on antiretroviral therapy and who develop serologic and clinical responses after treatment.

References

1. Rolfs RT, Joesoef MR, Hendershot EF, et al. A randomized trial of enhanced therapy for early syphilis in patients with and without human immunodeficiency virus infection. *N Engl J Med*. 1997;337(5):307–314.
2. Centers for Disease Control and Prevention. Neurosyphilis, ocular syphilis, and otosyphilis. 2021. Accessed June 13, 2023.https://www.cdc.gov/std/treatment-gui delines/neurosyphilis.htm
3. Workowski KA, Bachmann LH, Chan PA, et al. Sexually transmitted infections treatment guidelines, 2021. *MMWR Recomm Rep*. 2021;70(4):1–187.
4. Korenromp EL, Mahiané SG, Nagelkerke N, et al. Syphilis prevalence trends in adult women in 132 countries: Estimations using the Spectrum Sexually Transmitted Infections model. *Sci Rep*. 2018;8(1):11503.
5. Bowen VB, Braxton J, Davis DW, et al. Sexually transmitted disease surveillance 2018. National Prevention Information Network; 2019.
6. Korenromp EL, Rowley J, Alonso M, et al. Global burden of maternal and congenital syphilis and associated adverse birth outcomes: Estimates for 2016 and progress since 2012. *PLoS One*. 2019;14(2):e0211720.
7. Trivedi S, Williams C, Torrone E, Kidd S. National trends and reported risk factors among pregnant women with syphilis in the United States, 2012–2016. *Obstet Gynecol*. 2019;133(1):27–32.
8. Conde-Sendín MÁ, Amela-Peris R, Aladro-Benito Y, Maroto AA-M. Current clinical spectrum of neurosyphilis in immunocompetent patients. *Eur Neurol*. 2004;52(1):29–35.

29 "I Can't Concentrate Anymore"

Caleb R. S. McEntire and

Howard M. Heller

A 33-year-old woman with no significant medical history is referred to your clinic for fatigue. She reports to you that one year ago, she noticed a round, red rash on her left arm after hiking near her home in Connecticut. She presented to her PCP who diagnosed her with Lyme disease. She was treated with a full course of doxycycline, but since then she has noticed increasing fatigue. She used to hike 5 miles but now struggles to walk 1 or 2 miles. She also has difficulty concentrating, which has been impacting her work. You order an MRI of the brain, which is unremarkable, and blood work shows only 6/10 bands positive on Lyme IgG Western blot. She reports to you that she has been reading about chronic Lyme disease online, and she wonders if IVIG or IV ceftriaxone would be helpful in improving her condition.

What do you do now?

LYME DISEASE

Pathogenesis and Epidemiology

Lyme disease is an arthropod-borne virus (arbovirus) caused by species of the spirochete genus *Borrelia*, most commonly *B. burgdorferi* in the United States. It is carried by *Ixodes* ticks, which are distributed primarily throughout the Northeast and Midwestern United States and generally transmit disease during the eight-legged nymph stage of their life cycle, during which time they can be as small as 2 ml in length and so are usually not noticed by human hosts. The most common manifestations of the disease are rash and arthritis, but nervous system involvement can occur in 10–15% of symptomatic individuals. The stages of systemic disease can be divided into early localized, early disseminated, and late disease stages. Early localized Lyme disease is generally characterized by the appearance of the erythema migrans (EM) rash, which can appear with or without accompanying constitutional symptoms. Usually, EM emerges within 1 month following a tick bite. In this stage, the disease is limited to the site of infection.

Neurologic manifestations appearing during early disseminated Lyme disease include a characteristic triad of meningitis, facial nerve palsy, and radiculoneuritis, with this last manifestation also known as Bannwarth syndrome. Early disseminated Lyme disease occurs days to weeks after infection, manifesting as multiple EM lesions in up to half of patients. During this stage, spirochetes can spread and seed in the meninges. However, spread of spirochete from skin to the central nervous system (CNS) via peripheral nerves is likely responsible for at least some of CNS Lyme infection. In a study of 112 patients with Bannwarth syndrome compared to more than 12,000 patients with EM who did not experience neurological involvement, the patients with Bannwarth syndrome showed a significantly higher frequency of EM on their head, neck, and trunk. Furthermore, in 79% of these patients, the location of EM matched the dermatomes of radicular pain.[1]

Clinical Manifestations and Treatment

The most common CNS manifestation is a lymphocytic meningitis, which generally occurs weeks to months after the initial tick bite. This presents in a similar manner to meningitis due to other sources, with the caveat that nuchal rigidity can be absent or mild. In addition, cranial neuropathies can occur in up to 50% of patients with Lyme meningitis, which can be helpful in diagnosis before serum and cerebrospinal fluid testing have returned.

Bannwarth syndrome typically presents within weeks to months after initial Lyme disease infection, and it occurs in 3% of Lyme disease cases verified by the Centers for Disease Control and Prevention (CDC). Notably, nerve conduction studies on rhesus monkeys with Lyme disease have demonstrated mononeuropathy multiplex rather than a true radiculoneuritis, so it is possible that Bannwarth syndrome represents an entirely peripheral nervous system (PNS) disease or that elements of both CNS and PNS injury can contribute. This manifestation is less commonly diagnosed in the United States compared to meningitis or facial palsy, for instance.

Cardiac manifestations, most often atrioventricular block, and ocular manifestations such as conjunctivitis and uveitis can also occur during this stage. Some patients with early disseminated Lyme disease may not have a history of antecedent early localized Lyme disease.

Late Lyme disease is usually associated with intermittent or persistent arthritis that affects one or a few large joints, especially the knee, often preceded by migratory arthralgias. However, arthritis may be the first sign of the disease in some patients. Certain rare neurologic problems, primarily a subtle encephalopathy or polyneuropathy, may also develop months to a few years after the initial infection.

Lyme disease facial palsy (LDFP) is also relatively common, occurring in 9% of CDC-verified Lyme disease cases. This most commonly presents with unilateral, lower motor neuron pattern facial palsy, although bilateral facial palsy may be present in up to 20% of patients with LDFP. LDFP can be difficult to distinguish from Bell palsy (BP), but the treatment is notably different: Steroid administration worsens long-term outcomes of LDFP, whereas it improves outcome in BP.[2]

Lyme encephalitis is rare, occurring in approximately 3.3% of patients with Lyme neuroborreliosis. It presents with symptoms including altered mental status and cortical signs such as aphasia, ataxia, and seizures. MRI is poorly sensitive in this population, with findings consistent with encephalitis occurring only in approximately 20% of patients, although from the limited data available, electroencephalography appears to have abnormal findings in greater than 90% of patients.

Treatment for neurologic manifestations of Lyme disease specifically has been validated only in relatively small cohorts, so much of the treatment regimen is extrapolated from treatment of systemic Lyme. Oral doxycycline has been shown to be effective for LDFP and may be effective for Lyme meningoencephalitis and radiculitis as well,[3] but our practice is to use IV formulation of a third-generation cephalosporin, most often ceftriaxone, for these latter manifestations. Although there is no established gold standard for treatment duration, our practice is to use 14 days of oral doxycycline for patients with cranial nerve palsies only or 14 days of IV antimicrobial therapy for patients with meningoencephalitis.

Sex and Gender Differences in Lyme Manifestations

Although many sociocultural factors undoubtedly contribute to clinical manifestations of many pathogens, immune differences have also been clearly documented between sexes. Both sex and gender represent a spectrum, but for purposes of this discussion, we focus on the broad groups of male and female patients (often aligning with people assigned male and female at birth), which represent groupings of chromosomes, sex organs, and hormonal axes.

Women account for 80% of all diagnosed autoimmune disease in the United States, with varying ranges of intersex frequency documented both across and within individual diseases. Despite this, disease severity is approximately equal between sexes in most autoimmune conditions. The reason for this is not entirely clear. Hormonal differences may play a role; in animal models, female castration generally attenuates the severity of autoimmune disease, whereas male castration or estrogen supplementation worsens it. In human patients with multiple sclerosis, administration of testosterone was suggested to slow brain atrophy while modulating peripheral blood proxies of immune activation, although other studies have shown no effect of hormonal therapy on autoimmune disease in real clinical practice. Regardless of the specific effects of hormones, humoral responses to vaccines are generally more robust in women, as are both targeted and nontargeted post-vaccine reactions.

In Lyme disease specifically, there are sex differences in immune response and potentially clinical syndrome in acute Lyme infection between sexes. Males account for 56% of reported Lyme disease cases in the United States.

One study of 118 adult patients in Sweden found a significantly longer latency for EM resolution after treatment initiation in women compared to men, and significantly higher odds of developing non-annular skin lesions. Another study of 125 patients in the state of Maryland showed no clinical differences between male and female patients in systemic Lyme disease, but men had significantly higher numbers of enzyme-linked immunosorbent assay values and IgG bands compared to women. In a Slovenian study, men accounted for a majority of Lyme neuroborreliosis, but women accounted for the majority of diagnosed erythema migrans.

Regardless of pathophysiology, it is interesting to consider that given the more robust post-vaccine response in women, the post-infectious immune-mediated syndromes may also be more pronounced. However, both immunologic and sociocultural differences may play a role in post-infectious Lyme syndromes. Sex differences have been shown in infectious and post-infectious Lyme responses specifically. In one study of 142 Norwegian children diagnosed with Lyme neuroborreliosis, facial nerve palsy was significantly more common in female (86%) than in male patients (62%) (p < .001). The female patients in this study were younger than the male patients, had shorter symptom duration, and had a lower level of pleocytosis.[4]

It is also notable that in the United States, the incidence of documented Lyme disease is higher among whites than blacks which has often been attributed to higher exposure risks in white populations. However, underdiagnosis of the disease in people of color likely also plays a role at least in part because of underrecognition of erythema migrans on darker skin tones.

Post-Treatment Lyme Disease Syndrome

Post-treatment Lyme disease syndrome (PTLDS) refers to the presence of nonspecific symptoms that can persist for months after treatment of Lyme disease in approximately 5–15% of patients with Lyme disease.[5] These symptoms most commonly include fatigue, widespread musculoskeletal pain, and cognitive difficulties. A large meta-analysis in 2005 showed that these symptoms were present with 5% greater frequency in patients with PTLDS than in control populations without the disease, although the studies comprising this meta-analysis were unfortunately very heterogeneous in their definition of Lyme disease, with many patients diagnosed based on unreliable serologic testing such as nonspecific immunoblots. Many patients with nonspecific symptoms and positive Lyme serology are ultimately diagnosed with fibromyalgia, depression, or other underlying medical illnesses.

The pathophysiology that would underlie PTLSD as a primary entity is not entirely clear. Possibilities that have been proposed include decreased cerebral blood flow volume leading to diffuse cognitive deficits, but it is unlikely to involve persistent spirochete infection of the CNS.

Various diagnostic criteria have been proposed for classifying PTLDS,[6] with the common definitive criteria being a history of Lyme disease treated with an appropriate antimicrobial regimen and onset of systemic symptoms within a reasonable time frame to implicate infection as a cause (often within 6 months of initial Lyme infection). The terms *chronic Lyme* and *chronic Lyme disease* are used by some practitioners and many patients, although these terms do not have clear definitions.[5]

Our recommendations are that the diagnosis of PTLDS be used sparingly and that the 2006 Infectious Diseases Society of America (IDSA) diagnostic criteria be used strictly to rule in the diagnosis.[7] In addition, PTLDS diagnoses are often made in patients with no exposure to areas endemic for Lyme disease, which we recommend against. We do not recommend long-term parental antimicrobial therapy for patients with PTLDS because the risk and cost appear to outweigh the relatively slim potential benefits.[8]

Management of PTLDS is controversial, with no single gold standard of treatment. Some clinical trials using long-term IV antimicrobials (usually ceftriaxone) as an empiric therapy for disease have shown short-term or long-term benefits of the medications in terms of fatigue, but the adverse effects associated with ceftriaxone therapy generally outweighed any modest positive benefits. No trials have shown evidence for sustained improvement in specific PTLDS symptoms or overall quality of life with antimicrobial therapy compared to placebo that is sufficient to outweigh adverse effects. The most recent guidelines from IDSA recommend against IV or prolonged oral antibiotic therapy for cases of PTLDS.[7] IV immunoglobulin has essentially no evidence, either positive or negative, for treatment of PTLDS. Given the frequency of adverse effects with this therapy, and no evidence for benefit, it is not recommended to be used in PTLDS.[9] In general, the most effective treatment of PTLDS should be through identification and appropriate treatment of co-occurring pain, fatigue, or vertigo syndromes such as fibromyalgia, chronic regional pain syndrome, or postural orthostatic tachycardia syndrome.

KEY POINTS TO REMEMBER

- Neurologic manifestations of Lyme disease include meningitis, facial nerve palsy, and radiculoneuritis.
- Bell palsy should be distinguished from Lyme disease–related facial palsy because steroid treatment can worsen Lyme disease–related facial palsy.
- Lyme disease–related facial palsy can be treated with oral doxycycline, whereas other neurologic manifestations should be treated with 14–21 days of IV ceftriaxone.
- Post-treatment Lyme disease (chronic Lyme) does not have a clear treatment. An underlying cause, such as fibromyalgia, depression, chronic regional pain syndrome, or other primary cause of symptoms, should be identified and treated.

References

1. Ogrinc K, Kastrin A, Lotrič-Furlan S, et al. Colocalization of radicular pain and erythema migrans in patients with Bannwarth syndrome suggests a direct spread of *Borrelia* into the central nervous system. *Clin Infect Dis.* 2022;75(1):81–87.
2. Jowett N, Gaudin RA, Banks CA, Hadlock TA. Steroid use in Lyme disease–associated facial palsy is associated with worse long-term outcomes. *The Laryngoscope.* 2017;127(6):1451–1458.
3. Ljøstad U, Skogvoll E, Eikeland R, et al. Oral doxycycline versus intravenous ceftriaxone for European Lyme neuroborreliosis: A multicentre, non-inferiority, double-blind, randomised trial. *Lancet Neurol.* 2008;7(8):690–695.
4. Tveitnes D, Øymar K. Gender differences in childhood Lyme neuroborreliosis. *Behav Neurol.* 2015;2015:790762.
5. Feder HM Jr, Johnson BJ, O'Connell S, et al. A critical appraisal of "chronic Lyme disease." *N Engl J Med.* 2007;357(14):1422–1430.
6. Nemeth J, Bernasconi E, Heininger U, et al. Update of the Swiss guidelines on post-treatment Lyme disease syndrome. *Swiss Med Wkly.* 2016;146(4950):w14353.

7. Wormser GP, Dattwyler RJ, Shapiro ED, et al. The clinical assessment, treatment, and prevention of Lyme disease, human granulocytic anaplasmosis, and babesiosis: Clinical practice guidelines by the Infectious Diseases Society of America. *Clin Infect Dis*. 2006;43(9):1089–1134.

8. Fallon BA, Keilp JG, Corbera KM, et al. A randomized, placebo-controlled trial of repeated IV antibiotic therapy for Lyme encephalopathy. *Neurology*. 2008;70(13):992–1003.

9. Wong KH, Shapiro ED, Soffer GK. A review of post-treatment Lyme disease syndrome and chronic Lyme disease for the practicing immunologist. *Clin Rev Allergy Immunol*. 2022;62(1):264–271.

30 COVID-19 Neurologic Complications During Pregnancy

Christina R. Catherine

A 32-year-old woman who is 32 weeks and 4 days gestation presents to the emergency department (ED) via ambulance after her friend found her minimally responsive, febrile, and having labored breathing. She is intubated en route to the hospital for poor respiratory status. The friend speaks to the ED physician and reports that the patient had recently been diagnosed with COVID-19. She has a history of hypertension, gestational diabetes, and obesity. Neurological examination shows a somnolent woman who has no clear focal deficits when sedation is held. Basic lab work is notable for elevated creatinine, mild leukopenia, mild thrombocytopenia, normal liver function tests, and elevated urine protein:creatinine ratio. A discussion with the patient's spouse is held, with the recommendation for antenatal steroids and immediate cesarean section if the patient's condition worsens.

What do you do now?

COVID-19 INFECTION DURING PREGNANCY

Since September 2020, the World Health Organization (WHO) has warned pregnant people that they are at increased risk of severe COVID-19 infection, especially if they are older, overweight, or if they have preexisting medical conditions such as diabetes or hypertension.[1] This, in turn, can translate into an increased risk of maternal and neonatal morbidity and mortality.[2] Severe infections can lead to multiorgan dysfunction and require intubation with ventilatory support. In a Canadian study from March 1, 2020, through October 31, 2021, that examined the perinatal outcomes in 6,012 pregnant individuals diagnosed with SARS-CoV-2 infection, there was an increased risk of hospitalization in the pregnant patients versus non-pregnant women in the same age group (7.75% vs. 2.93%; 95% confidence interval [CI]: 2.41–2.88), increased risk of intensive care unit (ICU) admission (2.01% vs. 0.37%; 95% CI: 4.50–6.53), and increased risk of preterm birth (11.05% vs. 6.76%; 95% CI: 1.52–1.76).[3] Another study early in the COVID pandemic summarized case reports of neurological complications and COVID-19 infection in 18 women during the alpha or delta waves.[1] It found that half of the patients had central nervous system (CNS) disease, ranging from stroke to cerebral venous sinus thrombosis, posterior reversible encephalopathy syndrome (PRES), acute CNS demyelination, and acute necrotizing encephalopathy. In this cohort, maternal complications included a high ICU admission rate (approximately 50%) and high cesarean section rate (64.7%), whereas neonatal complications included three intrauterine fetal demises (16.67%). An interesting finding of this report was a high rate of reported new-onset hypertension without a clear diagnosis of comorbid preeclampsia given.

A reply to the previously discussed study noted two additional pregnant patients who developed Guillain–Barré syndrome (GBS) and one who developed large-vessel occlusion not included in the review. The first patient with GBS was a 29-year-old primigravida woman at 18 weeks of gestation with mild COVID-19 who developed length-dependent sensory and motor deficits and was found by nerve conduction studies (NCS) to have GBS. She had good recovery after administration of intravenous immunoglobulin (IVIG). The second was a 32-year-old woman in her eighth month of gestation admitted for headache, paresthesias, and ultimately quadriparesis in the context of SARS-CoV-2 positivity on admission. She received emergency cesarean section and soon thereafter developed bradycardia and respiratory insufficiency requiring mechanical ventilation. She was diagnosed with GBS by NCS and had incomplete recovery after IVIG administration. A third patient, an 18-year-old woman at 7 weeks of gestation, experienced sudden-onset left hemiparesis due to right middle cerebral artery infarct. She arrived out of the time frame for acute interventions but had incomplete recovery with dual antiplatelet therapy.

Another case report describes development of GBS following delivery in a pregnant woman. A 34-year-old woman at 37 weeks and 4 days gestation presented with COVID-19 symptoms and received cesarean section, and 16 days later she reported to the emergency room. Other case reports of GBS in pregnancy include a 22-year-old woman who developed length-dependent sensory and motor deficits and had GBS diagnosis confirmed by NCS. She was treated with IVIG with good effect.[4] Multiple case reports have also described acute inflammatory demyelinating polyneuropathy variants with facial diplegia in the context of pregnancy. It is difficult to draw a causal link in these cases between pregnancy and manifestations of GBS, but providers should consider that pregnancy and delivery may exacerbate existing manifestations of the disease or possibly contribute to precipitation of the disease after COVID-19.

COVID-19 infection during pregnancy has also been associated with an increased risk of developing a hypertensive disorder of pregnancy (HDP; odds ratio: 3.68).[5] HDP can have significant potential impacts to both the mother and her fetus. There is a known increased risk of preterm birth, intrauterine growth restriction, miscarriage, stillbirth, and increased maternal morbidity and mortality in pregnancies affected by HDP.[6] There are also long-term risks to the mother and the fetus. Infants who survive a pregnancy complicated by HDP are at increased risk for neurodevelopmental delay and complications of prematurity. Mothers who have had a pregnancy impacted by HDP are at increased risk of future stroke, myocardial infarction, and hypertension.[7] Diagnosis of HDP during pregnancy involves identifying systolic blood pressure greater than 140 mm Hg or diastolic blood pressure greater than 90 mm Hg with or without the presence of proteinuria as measured at least 4 hours apart.[8] Signs of end organ damage in the mother may also be present, including renal dysfunction, elevated liver function tests, thrombocytopenia, new-onset refractory headache, right upper quadrant pain, and pulmonary edema. Further discussion of this topic is explored in more detail in other chapters of this textbook.

Diagnosis of pregnancy-associated neurological complications in the setting of COVID-19 infection remains the same as that during the pre-COVID-19 era. Imaging with computed tomography (CT) of the head with appropriate shielding of the fetus is indicated if acute stroke is suspected. Magnetic resonance imaging (MRI) of the brain without contrast should be used in all other non-acute cases. CT angiography with contrast or diagnostic angiogram can be used with the caveat that fetal thyroid function would need to be monitored after birth and appropriate shielding should be used for the fetus. Blood work, including complete blood count, comprehensive metabolic panel with liver and renal function testing, and urine protein:creatinine ratio, should be obtained. Management of these neurologic complications is similar to that for patients without COVID-19 and should occur at a tertiary care center with access to maternal–fetal medicine, neonatology, and neurological services. Timing and mode of delivery should be determined by a multidisciplinary team on a case-by-case basis depending on the severity of infection, gestational age, and fetal status.

The risk of maternal morbidity/mortality and subsequently neonatal complications may have peaked during the 2021 delta variant wave. A report comparing perinatal outcomes between beta/delta waves and the omicron wave in Malawi was promising and showed lower rates of maternal morbidity or mortality with the omicron wave ($p \leq .05$), with only shortness of breath being associated with poor maternal outcomes ($p < .0001$).[9] The risk to mothers and their fetuses has also been altered by the availability of COVID-19 vaccinations that have proven to be safe and efficacious during pregnancy at protecting mothers from severe infections. These vaccines were available to the public starting in spring 2021 and recommended by obstetrical and midwifery organizations later that year as the delta wave peaked. The benefit of vaccination was demonstrated by data from Brazil which showed that pregnant women who were vaccinated had a 50% reduction in dyspnea and ICU admission, as well as an 80% reduction in intubation and maternal mortality, compared to unvaccinated pregnant women with COVID-19 infection.[9] The benefits of vaccination also extend to the fetus, likely through maternal antibody transmission, reducing the risk of COVID-19-related hospitalization and improving health outcomes after birth.[10]

In this case, the mother appears to have both severe COVID-19 infection and likely comorbid preeclampsia. She received a CT head at admission that was unremarkable but decompensated the day following admission, necessitating an emergency cesarean section for fetal distress and to help improve maternal oxygenation and respiratory compliance, as has been noted in studies prior to COVID-19. The infant required respiratory support at birth due to complications of prematurity and was discharged in healthy condition from the neonatal intensive care unit 7 weeks later. The mother's respiratory status improved following delivery, but she was noted to have cortical blindness and generalized seizure; MRI brain showed signs of PRES. Her blood pressure was treated appropriately, and her neurological symptoms slowly improved. Her hospital course was further complicated by a deep vein thrombosis and pulmonary embolus requiring anticoagulation. She was able to be discharged home neurologically intact approximately 3 weeks after admission.

KEY POINTS TO REMEMBER

- COVID-19 infection in pregnancy has the potential for significant morbidity or mortality for both the mother and the fetus, depending on the severity of the illness.
- Hypertensive disorders of pregnancy should be rapidly identified and treated to prevent harm and potential morbidity/mortality for the mother and fetus. These are more common in women who have or have had COVID-19 infection during pregnancy.
- Neurological complications can arise during pregnancy in relation to concurrent COVID-19 infection.
- The mode of delivery should be determined on a case-by-case basis depending on the status of the mother and the fetus, the gestational age of the fetus, and with the help of a multidisciplinary care team.

References

1. Magalhães JE, Sampaio-Rocha-Filho PA. Pregnancy and neurologic complications of COVID-19: A scoping review. *Acta Neurol Scand*. 2022;146(1):6–23.

2. Smith ER, Oakley E, Grandner GW, et al. Perinatal COVID PMA Study Collaborators. Adverse maternal, fetal, and newborn outcomes among pregnant women with SARS-CoV-2 infection: An individual participant data meta-analysis. *BMJ Global Health*. 2023;8:e009495.

3. McClymont E, Albert AY, Alton GD, et al. Association of SARS-CoV-2 infection during pregnancy with maternal and perinatal outcomes. *JAMA*. 2022;327(20):1983–1991.

4. Garcia JJ, Turalde CW, Bagnas MA, Anlacan VM. Intravenous immunoglobulin in COVID-19 associated Guillain–Barré syndrome in pregnancy. *BMJ Case Rep*. 2021;14(5):e242365.

5. Baracy M Jr, Afzal F, Szpunar SM, et al. Coronavirus disease 2019 (COVID-19) and the risk of hypertensive disorders of pregnancy: A retrospective cohort study. *Hypertens Pregnancy*. 2021;40:226–235.

6. Metz TD, Clifton RG, Hughes BL, et al. Association of SARS-CoV-2 infection with serious maternal morbidity and mortality from obstetric complications. *JAMA*. 2022;327:748–759.

7. Miller EC, Miltiades A, Pimentel-Soler N, et al. Cardiovascular and cerebrovascular health after pre-eclampsia: The Motherhealth prospective cohort study protocol. *BMJ Open*. 2021;11(1):e043052. doi:10.1136/bmjopen-2020-043052

8. Karrar SA, Martingano DJ, Hong PL. Preeclampsia. In: *StatPearls* [Internet]. StatPearls Publishing; 2023. https://www.ncbi.nlm.nih.gov/books/NBK570611

9. Costa ML, Charles CM. COVID-19 in pregnancy: Evidence from LMICs. *Lancet Global Health*. 2022;10(11):E1545–E1546.

10. Rasmussen SA, Jamieson DJ. COVID-19 vaccination during pregnancy—Two for the price of one. *N Engl J Med*. 2022;387(2):178–179.

SECTION VII

Neuro-Oncology

31 Newlywed With Headache, Morning Sickness, and Right-Sided Weakness

Varun Jain and Kevin B. Elmore

A 26-year-old woman presented to her PCP with a 2-month history of progressively worsening headaches that are worse upon awakening with increasing episodes of nausea, fatigue, and right arm weakness. She initially attributed her symptoms to stress and poor diet. No changes in vision, speech, mentation, or gait. Contrasted head CT was concerning for a left cerebral mass. The patient was sent for a brain MRI and referred to the neuro-oncologist for further evaluation (Figure 31.1). On examination, the patient was tachycardic and appeared visibly anxious. She had bilateral papilledema, slight right facial droop, decreased acuity in the right visual field, and decreased strength in the right hemibody. The remainder of the examination was unremarkable. The neuro-oncologist begins to discuss the most likely diagnosis and next steps. Overwhelmed, the patient interrupts, "But my husband and I are planning to start a family!"

What do you do now?

CANCER TREATMENTS AND FERTILITY PRESERVATION

Thalamic Glioblastoma, Limited Treatment Options, and Family Planning

The early signs of a brain tumor may be vague, intermittent, and less likely to prompt patients who are often otherwise healthy to seek immediate medical attention. Progression of undiagnosed brain tumors may lead to more advanced presentations and negatively influence outcomes. Reports of worsening headaches, focal neurological deficits, and occupational disability are more likely to lead to brain imaging. The presence of a heterogeneously enhancing mass with surrounding hyperintensity should raise concerns for a high-grade primary brain tumor. In this case, she was ultimately diagnosed with glioblastoma.

Glioblastoma is an aggressive and incurable brain malignancy with a median survival of 15 months. Management involves surgical resection, radiotherapy, and chemotherapy. Fertility may be affected by these treatments depending on patient characteristics, including age and sex, the anatomical location of the tumor, radiotherapy intensity and fields, and the route and duration of chemotherapy. Tumors involving the hypothalamic–pituitary region may result in hormonal dysregulation impacting fertility through the direct compressive effects of the tumors or detrimental effects of surgery and radiation therapy.[1] Alkylating agents, such as temozolomide, are commonly used chemotherapeutic drugs for primary brain tumors. Exposure to this drug class can potentially result in progressive, irreversible damage to the ovaries leading to premature ovarian failure.[2]

The patient should be informed of her risk of treatment-related infertility and offered referral to a reproductive specialist for discussion of fertility preservation options before starting treatment. This assessment should include discussions of baseline fertility, options for fertility preservation, and issues surrounding pregnancy with cancer. Standard methods for fertility preservation include oocyte preservation, embryo preservation, and ovarian tissue preservation.[3] Despite many studies indicating that patients desire counseling about fertility issues, women continue to be underinformed about fertility preservation options. Concerns surrounding delays in treatment while undergoing fertility preservation should be handled on a case-by-case basis while considering the aggressiveness of the disease.

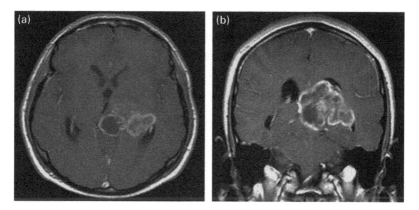

FIGURE 31.1 Magnetic resonance imaging of the brain, T1-weighted post-contrast images. Enhancing lesion of left thalamus on axial (a) and coronal (b) views with noted mass effect on surrounding brain structures.

Photo courtesy of Dr. Steven Toms, Neurosurgeon.

Pregnancy results in hemodynamic and hormonal changes that may influence brain tumor growth. Women are more than twice as likely to develop nonmalignant meningioma, suggesting hormonal influences associated with estrogen and progesterone receptors that are present on most meningiomas.[4] There are conflicting studies on oral contraception, hormone therapy, and pregnancy-associated meningioma growth, including reports of dramatic meningioma growth during pregnancy.[5] Population-based studies have both supported and refuted pregnancy as a risk factor for developing meningioma. Similarly, tumor progression has been observed in women with glioma during pregnancy, but larger studies to confirm these findings are lacking.

Management of brain tumors during pregnancy requires a multidisciplinary approach involving experienced providers from oncology, obstetrics, and neonatology. Neurosurgical procedures and the use of general anesthesia during pregnancy have been associated with risks of miscarriage and prematurity.[6] Safest surgical techniques involve carefully planned operative positioning and fetal monitoring. Radiation therapy is teratogenic and requires appropriate precautions to minimize the dose of scattered radiation reaching the fetus, such as use of a shielding device.[7] Certain forms of chemotherapy have been shown to cross the placenta with the potential to negatively impact fetal development, resulting in spontaneous abortion, fetal death, and malformation. Contraception is recommended in reproductive age women during treatment to avoid unintentional pregnancy and exposure to the potentially harmful effects of cancer treatments. Risks to the fetus are typically highest with organogenesis during the first trimester. In appropriate cases, these risks may be reduced by delaying treatments until after the first trimester, and preferably after delivery in stable patients.[8]

In summary, delays in diagnosis and initiation of treatment are common hurdles in cancer care. Despite pressures for the timely initiation of therapy, clinicians must counsel patients regarding treatment impacts on fertility and options for fertility preservation. Holistic treatment plans will inform patients of their diagnosis and treatment strategies while also addressing patient concerns surrounding family planning.

KEY POINTS TO REMEMBER

- Brain tumor treatments may negatively impact fertility. Fertility preservation, family planning, and pregnancy prevention should be discussed prior to the initiation of treatment.
- Standard methods for fertility preservation include oocyte preservation, embryo preservation, and ovarian tissue preservation.
- Management of brain tumors during pregnancy is complex and requires a multidisciplinary approach involving experienced providers from oncology, obstetrics, and neonatology.

References

1. Marques JVO, Boguszewski CL. Fertility issues in aggressive pituitary tumors. *Rev Endocr Metab Disord.* 2020;21(2):225–233. doi:10.1007/s11154-019-09530-y
2. Molina JR, Barton DL, Loprinzi CL. Chemotherapy-induced ovarian failure: Manifestations and management. *Drug Saf.* 2005;28(5):401–416. doi:10.2165/00002018-200528050-00004
3. Roberts JE, Oktay K. Fertility preservation: A comprehensive approach to the young woman with cancer. *J Natl Cancer Inst Monogr.* 2005;(34):57–59. doi:10.1093/jncimonographs/lgi014

4. Ostrom QT, Price M, Neff C, et al. CBTRUS statistical report: Primary brain and other central nervous system tumors diagnosed in the United States in 2016–2020. *Neuro Oncol.* 2023;25(12 Suppl 2):iv1–iv99. doi:10.1093/neuonc/noad149

5. Lusis EA, Scheithauer BW, Yachnis AT, et al. Meningiomas in pregnancy: A clinicopathologic study of 17 cases. *Neurosurgery.* 2012;71(5):951–961. doi:10.1227/NEU.0b013e31826adf65

6. Devroe S, Bleeser T, Van de Velde M, et al. Anesthesia for non-obstetric surgery during pregnancy in a tertiary referral center: A 16-year retrospective, matched case–control, cohort study. *Int J Obstet Anesth.* 2019;39:74–81. doi:10.1016/j.ijoa.2019.01.006

7. Kal HB, Struikmans H. Radiotherapy during pregnancy: Fact and fiction. *Lancet Oncol.* 2005;6(5):328–333. doi:10.1016/S1470-2045(05)70169-8

8. van Westrhenen A, Senders JT, Martin E, DiRisio AC, Broekman MLD. Clinical challenges of glioma and pregnancy: A systematic review. *J Neurooncol.* 2018;139(1):1–11. doi:10.1007/s11060-018-2851-3

SECTION VIII

Neuro-Ophthalmology

32 A Woman With Painful Blurry Vision

Islam Zaydan

A 28-year-old female presents to the ED with acute onset of blurred vision in her right eye. Her symptoms started about 24 hours ago and worsened over the past 6 hours. She describes the blurry vision as a cloud covering the center of her vision. She has aching pain with lateral eye movements. She denies any recent trauma, weakness, sensory changes, headache, dysphagia, dysarthria, or imbalance. She has no PMH and no family history of ocular or neurologic conditions. She denies tobacco, alcohol, or drug use. On examination, vital signs were normal. Neurologic examination showed the following right eye deficits: decreased visual acuity, color desaturation, an afferent pupillary defect, and a central visual field defect. A noncontrast head CT was negative; however, brain MRI revealed acute retrobulbar optic neuritis (Figure 32.1).

What do you do now?

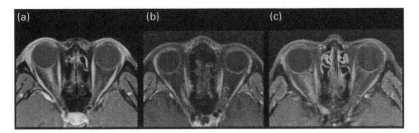

FIGURE 32.1 The majority of cases (67%) affect females usually 20–40 years of age, with higher incidence in the northern latitudes. In the United States, the incidence is estimated to be 6.4 per 100,000, and ON is commonly associated with MS. In Asia, ON is proportionately more common than MS: 90% of cases are monocular, with 10% binocular presentation common in children and Asian and African Americans.

OPTIC NEURITIS

Optic neuritis (ON) is an inflammatory, demyelinating condition affecting the optic nerve(s). It is commonly associated with other demyelinating conditions of the central nervous system (CNS), namely multiple sclerosis (MS). ON is a common presenting symptom of MS in 15–20% of cases.[3] Also, 50% of patients with MS will experience an attack of ON during their life with the disease. Thirty percent of patients will have inflammation of the optic disc (papillitis), with 67% of cases having retrobulbar inflammation.[4]

Pathologically, ON is caused by the infiltration of the optic nerve with pro-inflammatory cells and the excretion of cytokines, leading to edema followed by breakdown of the myelin sheath. Histologically, perivascular cuffing, edema, and eventual degradation of the myelin sheath are noted. Systemic activation of T cells and later B cells has been typically noted preceding clinical presentation.[7] Genetic susceptibility is suspected and is currently supported by an overrepresentation of certain human leukocyte antigen (HLA) subtypes in some patients.[9]

ON remains a clinical diagnosis supported by the constellation of symptoms (visual field defect—usually a central scotoma, color desaturation, ocular pain exaggerated with eye movements, afferent pupillary defect, and possible retinal changes) supported by the magnetic resonance imaging (MRI) findings. Evaluation should include detailed neurologic and ophthalmic history and examination. Laboratories include inflammatory markers (sedimentation rate and C-reactive protein), mimickers of demyelinating diseases (Sjogren disease, sarcoidosis, systemic lupus erythematosus, neuromyelitis optica [NMO], and anti-myelin oligodendrocyte glycoprotein [MOG] antibody) and, in certain cases, infectious etiologies (Lyme, varicella zoster virus, herpes simplex virus, syphilis, *Bartonella*, and HIV). In the majority of cases, ON is a monocular phenomenon; however, in 20% of cases, findings in the contralateral eye are found during the initial workup. These findings include visual acuity decline, contrast and color perception decline, visual field defects, as well as visual testing abnormalities. Brain MRI with and without contrast of the brain and orbits, preferably with fat suppression, is crucial in confirming the diagnosis and evaluating the risk of development of CNS demyelinating conditions. Spine MRI (cervical and thoracic) with and without contrast should also be performed in cases suspicious for MS and NMO. Cerebrospinal fluid (CSF) analysis for basic chemistry, cell counts, MS panel, CSF cytology, and Lyme serology are helpful in certain cases.[8] Glial fibrillary acidic protein astrocytopathy may cause ON (frequently papillitis). Patients may present with encephalopathy, headache, or transverse myelitis. The MRI brain shows a unique pattern of linear radial enhancement along the perivascular vessels, perpendicular to the lateral ventricles; workup and treatment of this distinct cause of ON are discussed elsewhere in this volume.

Visual field testing and ocular coherence tomography (OCT) are helpful tests to support the diagnosis and monitor the recovery. Typical visual field defects are central scotomas, paracentral scotoma, and arcuate defects. OCT outlines the swelling pattern of the optic disc and the retina, as well as the atrophy of the retinal nerve fiber layer that follows. OCT also helps diagnose retinal or macular conditions that could simulate ON.[2] Fluorescein angiography is used when suspecting a retinal condition, and it may show vascular sheathing and perivascular edema. These findings point to an increased risk of MS.[6] Visual evoked potentials (VEPs) can also be checked; in the case of ON, they will show unilateral delay in the P-100 wave. Multifocal VEP is more sensitive and specific in detecting ON cases.

Treatment

The standard of care treatment is 1,000 mg intravenous (IV) methylprednisolone for 3–5 days, sometimes followed by an oral steroid taper until 14 days of treatment if completed (Optic Neuritis Treatment Trial).[1] The use of IV steroids compared to oral steroids or placebo led to a more rapid recovery of vision, but there was no statistically significant difference in the long-term outcome with respect to visual acuity, visual fields, and color/contrast perception. IV steroids versus oral steroids had twice the rate of recurrent ON in the 6 months following treatment.[5] Other treatment options include IV immunoglobulin (IVIG) or plasmapheresis in patients who fail to respond to steroid therapy. Plasmapheresis is the preferred treatment modality in patients with NMO or MOG-associated disease diagnoses. ON treatment during pregnancy should be approached with caution because the use of high doses of steroids during certain stages of pregnancy may cause long-term complications for the fetus. In these circumstances, the use of alternative modalities of treatment (IVIG or plasmapheresis) should be considered. In patients who are recently postpartum and breastfeeding, IV steroids may be divided int oequal doses over 4 days to lower the daily dose, followed by an oral steroid taper.

Good recovery is expected in 97% of patients; poor recovery is noted in the remaining patients, who often present with severe visual loss, long segment of enhancement on the brain MRI, absent P-100 on the VEP, and are NMO antibody positive. Recovery can take up to 1 year. ON has a strong relationship to CNS demyelinating conditions, and neurology follow-up with these patients with appropriate imaging and clinical examination should occur. The risk of conversion to clinically definite MS after a single attack of ON remains high: 19% in cases with no white matter changes on the brain MRI and 51% in patients who show white matter demyelinating plaques on the initial MRI.

KEY POINTS TO REMEMBER

- Optic neuritis presents with painful vision loss or obscuration (blurriness, color desaturation, and central scotoma) that presents acutely and can last for days to weeks.
- Ruling out infectious or autoimmune mimics is necessary before starting treatment to confirm diagnosis.
- Treatment consists of high-dose IV steroids; in select circumstances, IVIG or plasmapheresis may also be used.
- Close follow-up with neurology and neuro-ophthalmology should be arranged for all patients.

References

1. Beck RW. The Optic Neuritis Treatment Trial. *Arch Ophthalmol.* 1988;106:1051–1053.

2. de Seze J, Blanc F, Jeanjean I, et al. Optical coherence tomography in neuromyelitis optica. *Arch Neurol.* 2008;65:920–923.

3. Francis DA, Compston DA, Batchelor JR, McDonald WI. A reassessment of the risk of multiple sclerosis developing in patients with optic neuritis after extended follow-up. *J Neurol Neurosurg Psychiatry.* 1987;50(6):758–765.

4. Frohman EM, Frohman TC, Zee DS, McColl R, Galetta S. The neuro-ophthalmology of multiple sclerosis. *Lancet Neurol.* 2005;4(2):111–121.

5. Sellebjerg F, Nielsen HS, Frederiksen JL, Olesen J. A randomized, controlled trial of oral high-dose methylprednisolone in acute optic neuritis. *Neurology.* 1999;52(7):1479–1484.

6. Lightman S, McDonald WL, Bird AC, et al. Retinal venous sheathing in optic neuritis: Its significance for the pathogenesis of multiple sclerosis. *Brain.* 1987;110(Pt 2):405–414.

7. Roed H, Frederiksen J, Langkilde A, Sørensen T, Lauritzen M, Sellebjerg F. Systemic T-cell activation in acute clinically isolated optic neuritis. *J Neuroimmunol.* 2005;162:165–172.

8. Söderström M, Link H, Xu Z, Fredriksson S. Optic neuritis and multiple sclerosis: Anti-MBP and anti-MBP peptide antibody-secreting cells are accumulated in CSF. *Neurology.* 1993;43:1215–1222.

9. Frederiksen J, Madsen H, Ryder L, Larsson H, Morling N, Svejgaard A. HLA typing in acute optic neuritis: Relation to multiple sclerosis and magnetic resonance imaging findings. *Arch Neurol.* 1997;54:76–80.

33 Painless Loss of Vision

Islam Zaydan

A 65-year-old woman presented with acute onset of painless loss of the inferior portion of the visual field of her left eye. Her visual symptoms were preceded by a mild periocular pain that resolved with the onset of the visual symptoms. She did not endorse any current headaches, polymyalgia rheumatica symptoms, jaw pain, recurrent oral ulcerations, or weight loss. She was noted to have elevated systolic blood pressure. Neurologic examination was unremarkable. Ophthalmic examination showed a decrease in the visual acuity: 20/20 right eye, 20/80 left eye. She had the following left eye deficits: decreased color saturation, an afferent pupillary defect, and an inferior altitudinal visual field defect. Fundus examination showed hyperemia of the optic disc with a small cup to disc ratio, sectoral edema of the superior portion of the optic disc, and a small flame hemorrhage at the disc margin (Figure 33.1). Noncontrast head CT was negative. CBC, ESR, and CRP were normal.

What do you do now?

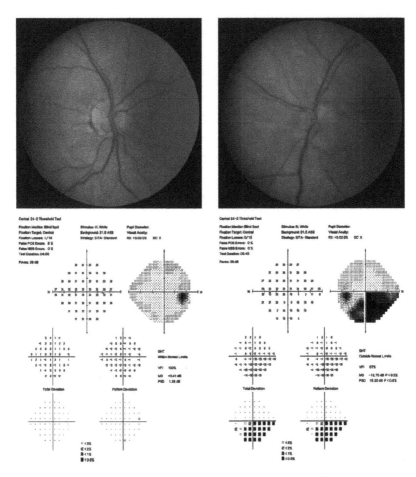

FIGURE 33.1 Fundus examination shows hyperemia of the left optic disc with a small cup to disc ratio, sectoral edema of the superior portion of the left optic disc, and a small flame hemorrhage at the left optic disc margin. Fundus photos and Humphrey visual field testing shows the sectoral left optic disc edema and the left inferior altitudinal visual field defect.

ACUTE ISCHEMIC OPTIC NEUROPATHY

Ischemic optic neuropathy (ION) is a vascular condition caused by occlusion of the retrobulbar ciliary arteries leading to ischemic damage to the optic nerve(s).[1] It typically affects patients older than age 50 years, with a male predominance, particularly in patients with underlying vascular risk factors. Incidence is estimated to be 11.3 per 100,000. It comprises three clinical entities: non-arteritic anterior ischemic optic neuropathy (NAION), posterior ischemic optic neuropathy (PION), and arteritic ischemic optic neuropathy (AION; commonly associated with giant cell arteritis).[1] Classic presentation is painless, monocular visual loss affecting a portion of the visual field with associated "altitudinal defects or arcuate defects." Occasionally, presentation is preceded by subtle periocular pain. The visual field loss may progress within the first 2 weeks, followed by stability and occasional improvement.

The diagnosis of ION is a clinical diagnosis, typically reached with the constellation of symptoms suggestive of optic neuropathy: decrease in visual acuity, decrease in brightness and color perception, afferent pupillary defect, and a visual field defect. The onset is typically acute with no preceding headache or other neurological deficit. Ophthalmic examination findings show signs of "disc at risk" with small cup:disc ratio, crowded optic disc, and may reveal arteriolar attenuation, as well as a sectoral optic disc edema and disc hemorrhage. Chronic hypertension, as well as other vascular risk factors, such as diabetes mellitus, hyperlipidemia, and smoking, have been implicated as causes of this vascular phenomenon. On pathology, lipohyalinosis of the short ciliary artery branches perfusing the optic nerve disc is seen in NAION. In PION, retrobulbar optic nerves are thought to be the cause of ischemia. AION has been linked to nocturnal hypotension caused by the use of high doses of antihypertensives at night, as well as the use of erectile dysfunction medications. PION has been linked to the same risk factors and is additionally associated with postsurgical procedures performed in the prone position or those with significant operative blood loss. Commonly, patients with PION will have similar presentation with the distinction of having normal fundus examination in many cases. The vision loss in AION is often more profound and may affect bilateral eyes.

It is of utmost importance to immediately obtain a detailed history, examination, and laboratories and to distinguish between NAION and AION (non-arteritic vs. arteritic origin). Findings suggestive of NAION instead of AION include the following[1]:

- Absence of polymyalgia rheumatica symptoms
- Lack of constitutional symptoms
- Lack of association with recurrent/new-onset headache

- Lack of symptoms suggestive of head/neck vascular ischemia
- The presence of multiple vascular disease risk factors
- Preserved visual acuity
- The presence of a disc at risk (small cup:disc ratio and a crowded disc)
- Findings of sectoral optic disc edema
- Normal systemic inflammatory markers, sedimentation rate, and C-reactive protein
- Lack of thrombocytosis and anemia
- Lack of profound optic disc atrophy on visual testing

Treatment and Prognosis

Unfortunately, there is currently no treatment for NAION that has been proven to change the course of the disease, improve visual outcome, or reduce the recurrence risk. Management of the hypertension gradually by avoiding hypotension that might exacerbate the ischemia and visual loss is recommended. Despite the vascular nature of NAION, antiplatelet therapy has not been proven to affect the visual outcome in clinical trials. Aspirin is usually recommended for patients after NAION because it has a secondary protective effect against cardiovascular disease and stroke.[7] Measures to avoid nocturnal hypotension are highly recommended (e.g., the use of morning anti-hypertensives instead of evening doses). When possible, medications that have been linked to NAION, such as phosphodiesterase-5 inhibitors, amiodarone, interferon-α, and sympathomimetics, should be discontinued given the potential for increasing the risk of contralateral eye involvement. Optic nerve sheath decompression surgery was previously studied but showed no benefit and, in fact, caused potential subsequent worsening of vision.[2,5,6,8] Vision restoration therapy is a new controversial vision rehabilitation modality with currently unproven benefit. Other associated vascular risk factors should be investigated and optimized, such as sleep apnea or hypercoagulable states. Temporal arteritis (giant cell arteritis) is discussed elsewhere in this textbook.

Patients with NAION often show worsening of the visual function within the first few weeks after onset, with eventual stabilization and rare improvement.[3] Significant disability is common in more than 50% of patients, with permanent visual acuity loss or restriction of the visual field; hence, visual rehabilitation and visual aids provided by low vision specialists are highly recommended.[4] Patients have a 5–7% risk of recurrence in the same eye and a 15–19% risk of recurrence in the contralateral eye. Diabetes and greater severity of NAION in the initially affected eye are risk factors for contralateral eye NAION. Risk of other vascular events, such as cardiac events or stroke, has not been noted after NAION.

KEY POINTS TO REMEMBER

- The classic presentation of non-arteritic anterior ischemic optic neuropathy (NAION) is acute, painless, and monocular vision loss affecting a portion of the visual field with associated altitudinal defects in an older patient with vascular risk factors.
- Ophthalmic examination reveals signs of an optic disc at risk with a small cup to disc ratio, crowded optic disc, sectoral optic disc edema, and disc hemorrhage.
- It is vital to distinguish between NAION and AION (non-arteritic vs. arteritic origin) because of differences in treatment.
- Unfortunately, there is currently no treatment for NAION that has been proven to change the course of the disease, improve visual outcome, or reduce the recurrence risk.
- Usual management includes blood pressure control and secondary prevention with aspirin.

References

1. Rucker JC, Biousse V, Newman NJ. Ischemic optic neuropathies. *Curr Opin Neurol.* 2004;17:27–35.
2. Characteristics of patients with nonarteritic anterior ischemic optic neuropathy eligible for the Ischemic Optic Neuropathy Decompression Trial. *Arch Ophthalmol.* 1996;114:1366–1374.
3. Arnold AC, Hepler RS. Natural history of nonarteritic anterior ischemic optic neuropathy. *J Neuroophthalmol.* 1994;14:66–69.
4. Hayreh SS, Zimmerman MB. Nonarteritic anterior ischemic optic neuropathy: Natural history of visual outcome. *Ophthalmology.* 2008;115:298–305.

5. Yee RD, Selky AK, Purvin VA. Outcomes of optic nerve sheath decompression for nonarteritic ischemic optic neuropathy. *J Neuroophthalmol.* 1994;14:70–76.

6. Scherer RW, Feldon SE, Levin L. Visual fields at follow-up in the Ischemic Optic Neuropathy Decompression Trial: Evaluation of change in pattern defect and severity over time. *Ophthalmology.* 2008;115:1809–1817.

7. Beck RW, Hayreh SS, Podhajsky PA, Tan ES, Moke PS. Aspirin therapy in nonarteritic anterior ischemic optic neuropathy. *Am J Ophthalmol.* 1997;123:212–217.

8. Newman NJ, Scherer R, Langenberg P, et al. The fellow eye in NAION: Report from the Ischemic Optic Neuropathy Decompression Trial Follow-up Study. *Am J Ophthalmol.* 2002;134:317–328.

34 New-Onset Headache With Vision Changes in an Elderly Woman

Islam Zaydan

A 73-year-old woman presented with 3 months of recurrent headaches and blurring of vision. The headaches are described as aching, affecting the vertex and temples, moderate to severe, not associated with nausea, vomiting, photophobia, or phonophobia, and unresponsive to NSAIDs. She also reported symptoms of polymyalgia rheumatica and jaw pain while chewing, and unintentional weight loss. She reported episodes of graying of the vision affecting both eyes, lasting for few minutes before resolving. Her vital signs showed systolic hypertension, mild tachycardia, and low-grade fever. Examination revealed generalized weakness with points of scalp tenderness. Fundus examination showed multiple hemorrhages on both optic discs and in the peripapillary area.

Basic labs revealed mild anemia, thrombocytosis, and elevated ESR and CRP.

Head CT was unremarkable. Brain MRI showed hyperintensity around the extracranial vessels with enhancement along the optic nerve sheaths.

What do you do now?

TEMPORAL ARTERITIS/GIANT CELL ARTERITIS

Giant cell arteritis (GCA; also known as Horton disease) is the most common type of systemic vasculitis. It affects the large and medium-size vessels and is most commonly seen in patients older than age 50 years, with a peak after age 70 years. Diagnosis of GCA should be suspected in patients who meet the following criteria[1,11]:

- Age older than age 50 years
- New-onset headache or an abrupt change in the preexisting headache semiology
- High ESR and CRP
- Visual changes (monocular or binocular amaurosis fugax)
- Jaw claudication
- Constitutional symptoms suggestive of polymyalgia rheumatica (unexplained fever, weight loss, nocturnal fever, and excessive sweating)[4]
- Vascular insufficiency symptoms (claudication, recurrent ulcerations, and tenderness along peripheral vessel courses)

The GCA risk calculator provided by the American College of Rheumatology can also be used[11]; scores ≥6 are strongly suggestive of GCA. If atypical features are present (lymphadenopathy, pulmonary infiltrates, large vessel cerebral infarction, mononeuritis multiplex, renal failure, or Raynaud phenomena), further investigation for other etiologies should be undertaken to rule out other causes, such as Takayasu arteritis or primary angiitis of the central nervous system, malignancy, or a systemic infection.

Diagnosis of GCA involves basic labs, vessel imaging, and temporal artery biopsy. Basic lab testing should include complete blood count, ESR, CRP, liver function tests, and albumin level. Elevated ESR and platelet count are most sensitive for helping identify patients at higher risk for GCA. Computed tomography angiograms of the neck and thoracic vessels (aorta and its branches) should be obtained, especially in cases with systemic symptoms.[10] Doppler ultrasound of the carotid, superficial temporal, and upper extremity arteries may be able to support the diagnosis of GCA in the future, but this is still an area of study.[3]

Diagnosis With Temporal Artery Biopsy

Urgent temporal artery biopsy should be performed but should not delay the initiation of steroid therapy once GCA is suspected. Temporal artery biopsy has a sensitivity range of 50–95%, with an average of 77.3% noted in clinical trials.[2] The sensitivity yield was noted in many clinical trials to decline linearly in relation to the length of stay with treatment and should generally not be performed after 4 weeks of steroid treatment. Up to 44% of patients with GCA may have false-negative results. Multiple factors increase the likelihood of false-negative results, including a "skip lesion" pattern of the histologic changes, the length of the biopsy, the number of histologic sections studied, and prolonged use of steroids prior to the biopsy. On histological examination, concentric rings of transmural infiltrates with inflammatory cells extending between the external and internal elastic lamina are present. Other pathological changes that may be present include laminar necrosis (in approximately 25% of cases), inflammatory changes of the adventitial layer sparing the intimal layers, intimal scarring, intimal hyperplasia, calcium deposition, and adventitious fibrosis; these have been noted in the chronic phase of the disease (Figure 34.1).

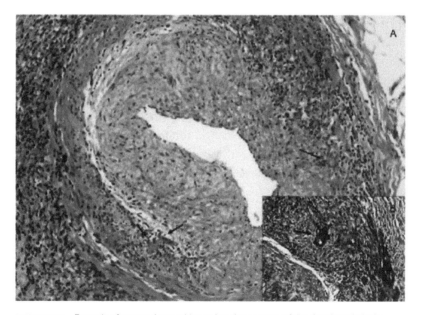

FIGURE 34.1 Example of temporal artery biopsy that shows some of the chronic pathologic changes of GCA including laminar necrosis, inflammatory changes of the adventitial layer sparing the intimal layers, intimal scarring, intimal hyperplasia, calcium deposition, and adventitious fibrosis.

Treatment

In cases of suspected GCA, high-dose glucocorticoids (e.g., prednisone 1 mg/kg or up to 60 mg daily or equivalent per European Alliance of Associations for Rheumatology guidelines or intravenous methylprednisolone 15 mg/kg for 3 days followed by oral prednisone taper if vision loss is already present per British Society for Rheumatology guidelines) should be initiated at the first patient encounter.[7] Steroids should be continued until a negative temporal artery biopsy result, or if there is still strong suspicion of GCA, repeat biopsy of the contralateral temporal artery should be performed. If GCA is confirmed on biopsy, prednisone should be continued at 60 mg daily for at least 1 month with clinical monitoring of symptoms (particularly vision) in conjunction with ESR/CRP marker normalization before tapering steroids. Treatment is continued for 12–18 months (up to 3 years) before tapering off glucocorticoids. Gastrointestinal prophylaxis with proton pump inhibitors and bone protection with calcium/vitamin D supplementation should be started simultaneously with steroid initiation.

To avoid the side effects and the risks of chronic high-dose glucocorticoid use, a steroid-sparing agent is highly recommended. Monoclonal interleukin-6 blocking antibody tocilizumab at 162 mg subcutaneous injection weekly or 6 mg/kg monthly infusion can be administered with glucocorticoids.[8,9] For patients with glucocorticoids and tocilizumab combined therapy, an accelerated glucocorticoid tapering regimen is followed, with cessation of steroids by 26 weeks. Methotrexate 10–15 mg weekly is an alternative steroid-sparing agent. For patients with symptoms of cerebral ischemia, the use of antiplatelet therapy in conjunction with glucocorticoids is recommended. For patients with vascular complications (organ/limb ischemia), revascularization procedures should be discussed along with vascular surgery. Several other steroid-sparing agents have efficacy in treating GCA; however, their use has not been widely adopted given the high risk of toxicity and limited data. These agents include abatacept, baricitinib, mavrilimumab, ustekinumab, azathioprine, leflunomide, dapsone, and cyclophosphamide.

Prognosis

Relapses are most prevalent in the first year of treatment, especially when trying to taper steroids. Relapses are suspected with reappearance of polymyalgia rheumatica symptoms, elevation in the inflammatory markers, cranial symptoms, or limb ischemia. Relapses during glucocorticoid monotherapy warrant increased dose or adding a steroid-sparing agent to the treatment regimen. Although remission is achieved in most patients within 1 or 2 years, a minority of patients might require low-dose therapy for longer duration.

KEY POINTS TO REMEMBER

- Giant cell arteritis is a medical emergency because patients can lose unilateral or bilateral vision.
- Steroid therapy should be immediately started to prevent vision loss.
- Temporal artery biopsy should be performed and repeated if GCA is still strongly suspected.
- Steroid-sparing agents may need to be used in cases with frequent relapses or significant side effects to chronic steroid therapy.

References

1. Hunsder GG, Bloch DA, Michel BA, et al. The American College of Rheumatology 1990 criteria for the classification of giant cell arteritis. *Arthritis Rheum.* 1990;33(8):1122–1128.
2. Rubenstein E, Maldini C, Gonzalez-Chiappe S, Chevret S, Mahr A. Sensitivity of temporal artery biopsy in the diagnosis of giant cell arteritis: A systematic literature review and meta-analysis. *Rheumatology.* 2020;59(5):1011–1020.
3. Schmidt WA, Kraft HE, Vorpahl K, Völker L, Gromnica-Ihle EJ. Color duplex ultrasonography in the diagnosis of temporal arteritis. *N Engl J Med.* 1997;337(19):1336–1342.
4. Buttgereit F, Dejaco C, Matteson EL, Dasgupta B. Polymyalgia rheumatica and giant cell arteritis: A systematic review. JAMA. 2016 Jun;315(22):2442–2458.
5. Bley, TA, Wieben O, Uhl M, Thiel J, Schmidt D, Langer M. High-resolution MRI in giant cell arteritis: Imaging of the wall of the superficial temporal artery *Am J Roentgenol.* 2005;184 (1):283–287.
6. Klink T, Geiger J, Both M, et al. Giant cell arteritis: Diagnostic accuracy of MR imaging of superficial cranial arteries in initial diagnosis—Results from a multicenter trial. *Radiology.* 2014;273:844–852.

7. Proven A, Gabriel SE, Orces C, O'Fallon WM, Hunder GG. Glucocorticoid therapy in giant cell arteritis: Duration and adverse outcomes. *Arthritis Rheum*. 2003;49:703–708.

8. Villiger PM, Adler S, Kuchen S, et al. Tocilizumab for induction and maintenance of remission in giant cell arteritis: A Phase 2, randomised, double-blind, placebo-controlled trial. *Lancet*. 2016;387:1921–1927.

9. Stone JH, Tuckwell K, Dimonaco S, et al. Trial of tocilizumab in giant-cell arteritis. *N Engl J Med*. 2017;377:317–328.

10. Prieto-González S, Depetris M, Gárcia-Martinez A, et al. Positron emission tomography assessment of large vessel inflammation in patients with newly diagnosed, biopsy-proven giant cell arteritis: A prospective, case–control study. *Ann Rheum Dis*. 2014; 73:1388–1392.

11. Ponte C, Grayson PC, Robson JC, et al.; DCVAS Study Group. 2022 American College of Rheumatology/EULAR classification criteria for giant cell arteritis. *Arthritis Rheumatol*. 2022;74(12):1881–1889. doi:10.1002/art.42325

SECTION IX

Movement Disorders

35 Parkinson's Disease in Women

Veronica Bruno and Elizabeth Slow

Ms. A, a woman in her early 50s, presented with a persistent, mild tremor in her right hand, which she had experienced for the last year. In addition to this tremor, she disclosed increased anxiety, which had begun to disrupt her daily life and overall well-being. Overnight, she struggled with insomnia and vivid, dreams. She struggled with chronic constipation and reduced sex drive. Concerned about these symptoms, Ms. A contacted her health care provider. She was referred to multiple specialists, and her symptoms were largely attributed to stress. Three years after persistently seeking answers, she saw a neurologist. On exam, Ms. A displayed a resting tremor in her right hand that diminished during purposeful movement. She also exhibited noticeable bradykinesia or slowness in initiating and executing movements, particularly in her right hand and fingers. Muscle rigidity was evident in her right arm and shoulder, leading to pain and a restricted range of motion.

What do you do now?

This case presents a constellation of symptoms that raise suspicion of Parkinson's disease (PD) in Ms. A. Although tremors are a hallmark motor symptom of PD, her non-motor symptoms, including anxiety, sleep disturbances, constipation, and diminished sexual desire, also align with the broader clinical spectrum of the disease. A comprehensive evaluation and medical assessment are warranted to confirm the diagnosis and initiate appropriate management and support.

PARKINSON'S DISEASE

Parkinson's disease is a progressive, neurodegenerative disorder that primarily affects movement. PD occurs when dopaminergic neurons begin to degenerate and die, leading to low levels of dopamine, a neurotransmitter necessary for smooth and coordinated muscle movement. Lewy bodies, composed of the protein alpha-synuclein, are the pathologic hallmark of PD. The underlying cause of PD is unknown, but it likely involves a combination of genetics and environmental factors. Most people who develop PD are older than age 60 years, and it is slightly more common in men than in women. PD is estimated at a prevalence of 1% of the population older than age 60 years. As more people live longer, the number of people with PD continues to increase throughout the world.[1]

The main motor symptoms of PD include slow movement (bradykinesia), muscle stiffness (rigidity), and a tremor that is present at rest. Balance (including falls) and walking are also affected, although usually later in the disease course. Non-motor symptoms are prominent and include cognitive and psychiatric changes, sleep disorders, and dysautonomia. Some of the non-motor symptoms predate the onset of motor symptoms by years or decades (often termed pre-motor symptoms) and include constipation, rapid eye movement (REM) sleep behavior disorder (in which patients act out their dreams), and olfactory loss. Diagnosis of PD is based on clinical history and examination—there are no confirmatory tests.[2] Treatment for PD involves symptom management as currently there are no disease-modifying therapies—that is, there is no way to slow or stop the disease progression (although there are many ongoing clinical trials for potential disease-modifying agents).

Diagnosis of Parkinson's Disease in Women

Parkinson's disease poses unique diagnostic and management challenges in women, who often face greater difficulty in obtaining a timely diagnosis compared to men.[3] Traditionally perceived as a condition primarily affecting older men, PD also affects many women throughout the world.[4] As mentioned previously, diagnosis typically hinges on clinical assessment, which involves evaluating the presence of resting tremor, bradykinesia, rigidity, and postural instability. Notably, in women, PD may manifest with subtler motor symptoms initially, adding complexity to the diagnostic process. Moreover, it is crucial to consider gender-specific factors, including hormonal influences.[5] Advanced diagnostic tools such as dopamine transporter imaging scans can be valuable in some cases, mainly for differentiating PD from other Parkinsonian syndromes, but they are not typically necessary for diagnostic confirmation.[2] Pregnancy in the context of PD presents additional challenges, as some women may experience exacerbated motor and non-motor symptoms while others report symptom stability; besides, careful medication management is essential since some antiparkinsonian drugs carry risks for birth defects, whereas levodopa is generally considered safe.

Management of Motor Symptoms

Following diagnosis, the management of motor symptoms is the focus of PD care. Commonly prescribed medications such as levodopa, dopamine agonists, and monoamine oxidase-B inhibitors play a pivotal role in treatment[1] (Table 35.1). Note that observations suggest that women may have a higher likelihood of experiencing medication-related dyskinesia, motor fluctuations, and wearing-off phenomena.[6] However, this could be because medication dosages and schedules in women may interact with hormonal changes during their menstrual cycle or menopause—an aspect of women's care that has not been extensively studied.

In addition to pharmacological interventions, physical therapy, occupational therapy, and exercise assume critical importance in enhancing mobility and reducing disability. In later stages, advanced therapies such as deep brain stimulation, subcutaneous or intestinal levodopa infusion can be considered.[7]

TABLE 35.1 Medications for Management of the Motor Symptoms of Parkinson's Disease

Medication	Dose	Adverse Effects	Comments
Dopamine Precursor			
Levodopa given with a peripheral decarboxylase inhibitor (carbidopa or benserazide)	Titrate to initial dose of 100/25 three times daily, maximum 1,500/375 mg/ day or more	Nausea/vomiting, orthostatic hypotension, dyskinesias, psychosis, motor fluctuations	Formulations Immediate release for any stage Controlled release: overnight akinesia Extended release (Rytary): treatment of motor fluctuations Levodopa–carbidopa intestinal gel: used with a pump for motor fluctuations
Dopamine Agonists			
Pramipexole	Start 0.125 mg three times daily, max 4.5 mg/day	Nausea, orthostatic hypotension, pedal edema, excessive sleepiness, impulse control disorder, psychosis	Early and adjunctive therapy Also available in an extended-release formulation
Ropinirole	Start 0.25 mg three times daily, max 24 mg/day	Same as pramipexole	Early and adjunctive therapy Also available as a prolonged-release formulation
Rotigitine (patch)	Start 2 mg/ 24 hr, max 16 mg/24 hr	Same as pramipexole Local skin reactions (dermatitis)	Early and adjunctive therapy Late therapy for motor fluctuations

TABLE 35.1 **Continued**

Medication	Dose	Adverse Effects	Comments
Apomorphine (parenteral)	3–5 mg SC injection PRN (or continuous infusion)	Same as pramipexole Local skin reactions (including nodules)	Late-stage motor fluctuations Requires concomitant antiemetic (e.g., domperidone)
Monoamine Oxidase B Inhibitors			
Selegiline	2.5 mg daily to 5 mg twice daily	Dopaminergic side effects of other drugs possibly accentuated, insomnia, confusion	Also available as a wafer formulation Last dose given at midday to avoid insomnia
Rasagiline	1 mg daily	Same as above	
Safinamide	50–100 mg daily		Used in conjunction with levodopa
Catechol-*O*-Methyltransferase Inhibitors			
Entacapone	200 mg with each dose of levodopa	Diarrhea in 5% Effects of levodopa accentuated	Adjunct only (with levodopa)
Opicapone	100 mg daily	As for entacapone	Adjunct only
Other			
Amantadine	100 mg to 300 mg daily	Peripheral edema, livedo reticularis, hallucinations, confusion	Anti-dyskinetic

Non-Motor Aspects of Parkinson's Disease in Women

Women with PD often experience a range of non-motor symptoms that significantly impact their quality of life. Anxiety and depression are prevalent, and addressing these mental health concerns is essential. Sleep disturbances, such as insomnia and vivid dreams, are common and may require medication or behavioral therapy. All these symptoms are more commonly reported in women.[7] Constipation, urinary urgency and frequency, sexual life changes, and symptoms of low blood pressure with position changes (orthostatic hypotension) are also common in PD.[8] In women, many of these symptoms may be mistaken for hormonal changes, such as those associated with menopause, making it more challenging to recognize them as part of PD and manage appropriately. Neuropsychiatric changes, including dementia and psychosis, can occur in later stage disease and lead to long-term care placement and increased mortality. See Table 35.2 for medication management of non-motor symptoms.

TABLE 35.2 **Medications for the Management of Non-Motor Symptoms of Parkinson's Disease**

Non-Motor Symptom	Medication	Dosing	Adverse Effects
Dementia	Cholinesterase inhibitors Donepezil Rivastigmine (oral or patch)	5–10 mg once daily 3–12 mg daily, patch: 4.5–9.8 mg/24 hr	Nausea, dizziness, headache
	NMDA antagonist Memantine	5–10 mg daily	Confusion, fatigue, dizziness, headache
Psychosis	Antipsychotic Clozapine Quetiapine	Start at 6.25–12.5 mg daily at bedtime; maximum 150 mg daily Start at 12.5–25 mg at bedtime; maximum 400 mg daily in divided doses	Sedation, orthostatic hypotension, sialorrhea, agranulocytosis Extrapyramidal symptoms and sedation

TABLE 35.2 **Continued**

Non-Motor Symptom	Medication	Dosing	Adverse Effects
	Inverse agonist/ antagonist serotonin 5-HT$_{2A}$ Pimavanserin	34 mg daily	Peripheral edema, confusion, nausea, constipation
	Cholinesterase inhibitor Rivastigmine	As above	As above
Depression and anxiety	Selective serotonin reuptake inhibitors Citalopram Fluoxetine Paroxetine Sertraline	10–20 mg once daily 10–50 mg once daily 20–40 mg once daily 20–200 mg once daily	Sexual dysfunction, anorexia, nausea, drowsiness
	Serotonin and norepinephrine reuptake inhibitor Venlafaxine	37.5–225 mg daily in divided doses	Sexual dysfunction, insomnia, drowsiness, gastrointestinal symptoms
Rapid eye movement sleep behavior disorder	Melatonin	3–15 mg nightly	Daytime sleepiness, headache, dizziness
	Clonazepam	0.25–2 mg nightly	Sedation and confusion
Orthostatic hypotension	Fludrocortisone	0.1–0.3 mg daily	Supine hypertension, hypokalemia
	Midodrine	2.5 mg daily up to 10 mg three times daily max	Supine hypertension
Constipation	Stimulant laxative Senna glycoside	Available in liquid, tablet, rectal suppository; for PRN usage	Abdominal pain/ cramps, nausea

(*Continued*)

TABLE 35.2 **Continued**

Non-Motor Symptom	Medication	Dosing	Adverse Effects
	Osmotic laxative Polyethylene glycol	Various formulations; can be used daily	Abdominal pain/ cramps, nausea, bloating, diarrhea
Urinary dysfunction	Mirabegron	25–50 mg	Headache, increased, blood pressure
Sialorrhea	Botulinum toxin	Dosage varies; parotid and/or submandibular glands	Dry mouth, dysphagia
Sexual dysfunction	Sildenafil	25–100 mg	Cardiac events, priapism, visual loss

Comprehensive Management and Patient-Centered Care

In the management of PD in women, adopting an integral, empowering, and patient-centered approach is of utmost importance. As the first step, it is crucial to acknowledge and address the distinct experiences and challenges that women with PD encounter. Treatment plans should be tailored to comprehensively address both the motor and non-motor aspects of the condition. Furthermore, the involvement of a multidisciplinary team, including, for example, neurologists, psychiatrists, physical therapists, and dietitians, can guarantee a well-rounded and comprehensive approach to care personalized to fit each patient's needs.

Conclusion

Parkinson's disease in women presents distinct diagnostic considerations and management challenges. Effective management encompasses addressing motor symptoms, tailoring medication regimens to account for hormonal fluctuations, and customizing the management of motor and non-motor symptoms through individually tailored interventions.

In the pursuit of optimal care for women with PD, fostering an empowering, patient-centered approach stands as a cornerstone to enhance their overall well-being and improve their quality of life.

KEY POINTS TO REMEMBER

- Parkinson's symptoms in women can initially be subtle, requiring careful clinical evaluation for diagnosis.
- Medication dosages may need adjustment due to hormonal fluctuations in women, particularly during the menstrual cycle and menopause.
- Management should encompass both motor and non-motor symptoms, including mental health support and addressing hormonal factors.
- A team of specialists, including neurologists, psychiatrists, and physical therapists, is crucial for comprehensive, patient-centered care.
- The goal is to enhance the overall well-being and quality of life of women with PD, recognizing their unique experiences and challenges.

References

1. Bloem BR, Okun MS, Klein C. Parkinson's disease. *Lancet.* 2021;397(10291):2284–2303. doi:10.1016/S0140-6736(21)00218-X
2. Subramanian I, Mathur S, Oosterbaan A, Flanagan R, Keener AM, Moro E. Unmet needs of women living with Parkinson's disease: Gaps and controversies. *Mov Disord.* 2022;37(3):444–455.
3. Postuma RB, Berg D, Stern M, et al. MDS clinical diagnostic criteria for Parkinson's disease. *Mov Disord.* 2015;30(12):1591–1601. doi:10.1002/mds.26424
4. Vaidya B, Dhamija K, Guru P, Sharma SS. Parkinson's disease in women: Mechanisms underlying sex differences. *Eur J Pharmacol.* 2021;895:173862.
5. Miller IN, Cronin-Golomb A. Gender differences in Parkinson's disease: Clinical characteristics and cognition. *Mov Disord.* 2010;25(16):2695–2703.
6. Umeh CC, Pérez A, Augustine EF, et al. No sex differences in use of dopaminergic medication in early Parkinson disease in the US and Canada: Baseline findings of a multicenter trial. *PLoS One.* 2014;9(12):e112287.
7. Picillo M, Amboni M, Erro R, et al. Gender differences in non-motor symptoms in early, drug naïve Parkinson's disease. *J Neurol.* 2013;260(11):2849–2855.
8. Chaudhuri KR, Schapira AH. Non-motor symptoms of Parkinson's disease: Dopaminergic pathophysiology and treatment. *Lancet Neurol.* 2009;8(5):464–474.

36 Huntington Disease

Jane Liao and Elizabeth Slow

A 45-year-old woman presents to your office with a 1½-year history of involuntary movements. Her husband has observed her becoming more "fidgety" initially during family gatherings but now nearly nightly. She has had a lifelong history of depression and dyslipidemia. She has been on long-term disability due to her mental health for the past 4 years. Her medications include escitalopram and rosuvastatin. Her family history is significant for Huntington disease (HD) in her paternal grandmother and alcohol use disorder in her father, who passed away from suicide.

On examination, she had a blood pressure of 132/67 mm Hg and pulse of 68 beats per minute. She made perseverative errors on Luria sequencing and scored 26/30 on the Montreal Cognitive Assessment test. She had slow saccades with suppressible head turns. She was unable to keep her tongue protruded for 10 seconds. She had choreiform movements affecting the face, head/neck, arms, and legs. Her gait is wide based but otherwise of normal speed and stride length. She stepped out twice on tandem gait but had a normal pullback test.

What do you do now?

Chorea, derived from the Greek word *chorós*, meaning dance, refers to involuntary, random, and nonrepetitive movements that can be seen in the face, trunk, and limbs. The movements are often continuous during wakefulness, disappear during sleep, and worsen during periods of stress. In the mild stages, chorea can appear like fidgeting to observers but commonly go unnoticed by patients themselves. In adults presenting with chronic chorea, the list of differential diagnoses can include autoimmune, paraneoplastic, toxic/nutritional, hematological, vascular, and genetic causes, but regardless of family history, it is pertinent to consider a diagnosis of HD.

HD is the most common cause of adult-onset hereditary chorea.[1] The average age of onset is in the fourth and fifth decades of life; however, 25% of patients develop symptoms after age 50 years.[2] The medial life expectancy is 15–20 years after symptom onset.[1] Affected patients develop a triad of movement disorders, cognitive impairment, and psychiatric/behavioral changes. In addition to chorea, other common motor manifestations include dysarthria, dysphagia, tics, parkinsonism, dystonia, and ataxia. In contrast, juvenile-onset HD (previously known as the "Westphal" variant) often presents with predominant parkinsonism and dystonia.[3] Seizures are also common.

Although the clinical diagnosis of HD is dependent on motor symptoms as evaluated by the Unified HD Rating Scale, cognitive and behavioral/psychiatric symptoms can be more detrimental to the patient and precede the diagnosis of HD (as determined by the onset of motor symptoms) by 10–15 years. Psychiatric/behavioral symptoms can range from depression and anxiety to addictions, psychosis, and increased risk of suicide. Cognitive symptoms are characterized by early impairment in attention and organization, with relative preservation of language function. Lack of insight, especially of one's own disabilities, is common.[2]

HD is caused by trinucleotide repeat expansion in the *huntingtin* (*HTT*) gene on chromosome 4 and inherited in an autosomal dominant fashion.[4] Children of HD patients have a 50% chance of inheriting the abnormal gene, but their clinical course, in part, depends on the length of CAG repeats. Patients with 40 or more repeats have full penetrance and are expected to become symptomatic in their lifetime. Patients with 36–39 repeats have reduced penetrance but can still develop the disease. Patients with 27–35 repeats are considered to be in the intermediate range, where patients do not develop clinical symptoms, but their children have a higher chance of developing HD. Patients with 26 or fewer repeats are considered to be in the normal range.[1] The number of CAG repeats is inversely correlated with the age of onset and severity of disease; however, it only accounts for 50–70% of the disease's overall variability.[3] Paternal anticipation is a well-defined phenomenon in HD such that children of an affected father can inherit a higher number of CAG repeats. Juvenile-onset HD with greater than 60 CAG repeats is also more commonly inherited from affected fathers than mothers.[2]

To diagnose HD, a thorough neurological assessment is required. Structural magnetic resonance imaging of the brain, particularly when performed early in the disease, can show focal caudate head atrophy.[5] Genetic testing is performed for confirmation. It is critical that patients receive the appropriate genetic counseling and support throughout the process. Asymptomatic children of HD patients should be allowed to make an informed decision whether to pursue testing once they reach the appropriate age for consent. Counseling around family planning is also important for known asymptomatic carriers and ideally done before a pregnancy. Prenatal testing is available for confirmed carriers through either chorionic villus sampling (11–13 weeks of gestation) or amniocentesis (14–18 weeks of gestation).[2] Alternatively, preimplantation genetic testing can provide direct testing of embryos obtained after in vitro fertilization with the intention to select unaffected embryos to be transferred into the uterus.[2]

Men and women are equally susceptible to develop HD, but natural history studies of HD have suggested there are sex differences in the disease course. Female HD patients present with worse motor, cognitive, and depression symptoms compared to males, but they have a lower frequency of alcohol misuse.[6]

To date, HD remains a neurodegenerative disease for which there is no cure. Management requires a multidisciplinary approach involving neurologists, psychiatrists, physiotherapists, occupational therapists, speech and language pathologists, dietitians, social workers, and genetic counselors. Patient resources and support groups can also be beneficial, particularly for newly diagnosed patients (Table 36.1).

TABLE 36.1 Huntington Disease Patient Resources

Huntington Society of Canada	https://www.huntingtonsociety.ca
Huntington's Disease Society of America	https://hdsa.org
International Huntington Association	https://huntington-disease.org
European Huntington's Disease Network	https://ehdn.org
HDBuzz	https://en.hdbuzz.net
National Institute of Neurological Disorders and Stroke: Huntington's Disease	https://www.ninds.nih.gov/health-information/disorders/huntingtons-disease

From Caron et al.[2]

The goal of pharmacological therapy in HD is to address symptoms and improve patients' quality of life. Therapies are individualized and based on expert consensus (Table 36.2). First-line treatment for chorea is vesicular monoamine transporter type 2 (VMAT2) inhibitors such as tetrabenazine, deutetrabenazine, and valbenazine.[4] Neuroleptics such as risperidone, olanzapine, and quetiapine are commonly used for patients with concurrent psychosis and chorea.[4] In pregnant women with HD, amantadine has been associated with fetal cardiac malformations.[7] The majority of neuroleptics and tetrabenazine are designated U.S. Food and Drug Administration pregnancy category C due to a lack of adequate studies.[7] In addition, exposure to neuroleptics in the third trimester has been associated with an increased risk of neonatal extrapyramidal symptoms.[8] In breastfeeding women with HD, it is known that both neuroleptics and tetrabenazine pass into the breast milk, but the infant risk is unclear.[7]

Although no disease-modifying therapy has yet been developed for HD, our collective understanding of HD has grown tremendously. Recently developed DNA and RNA targeting therapies aimed to reduce mutant HTT protein have shown promising results,[6]

TABLE 36.2 Selected Medications in Huntington Disease

Indication	Medication Class	Common Medication Choices
Chorea	VMAT2 inhibitors	Tetrabenazine, deutetrabenazine, valbenazine
	Neuroleptics	Risperidone, olanzapine, quetiapine
	NMDA receptor antagonist; increases dopamine release, blocks dopamine reuptake	Amantadine
Psychosis	Dopamine antagonists	Risperidone, olanzapine, quetiapine
Depression and anxiety	Selective serotonin reuptake inhibitor	Citalopram, sertraline
	Serotonin and noradrenaline reuptake inhibitor	Venlafaxine
	Presynaptic α_2 antagonist	Mirtazapine

KEY POINTS TO REMEMBER

- Huntington disease is the most common cause of adult-onset hereditary chorea.
- Cognitive and behavioral symptoms can be debilitating and precede HD diagnosis by up to 10–15 years.
- Paternal anticipation can lead to expanded CAG repeats and earlier age of onset in affected offspring.
- Tetrabenazine is the first-line symptomatic treatment for chorea in HD.

References

1. Stimming EF, Bega D. Chorea. *Continuum.* 2022;28(5):1379–1408.
2. Caron NS, Wright GEB, Hayden MR. Huntington disease. October 23, 1998. Updated June 11, 2020. In: Adam MP, Mirzaa GM, Pagon RA, et al., eds. *GeneReviews* [Internet]. University of Washington, Seattle; 2023. https://www.ncbi.nlm.nih.gov/books/NBK1305

3. Ross CA, Tabrizi SJ. Huntington's disease: From molecular pathogenesis to clinical treatment. *Lancet Neurol.* 2011;10(1):83–98.

4. Bachoud-Lévi AC, Ferreira J, Massart R, et al. International guidelines for the treatment of Huntington's disease. *Front Neurol.* 2019;10:710.

5. Stoker TB, Mason SL, Greenland JC, Holden ST, Santini H, Barker RA. Huntington's disease: Diagnosis and management. *Pract Neurol.* 2022;22(1):32–41.

6. Hentosh S, Zhu L, Patino J, Furr JW, Rocha NP, Furr Stimming E. Sex differences in Huntington's disease: Evaluating the Enroll-HD database. *Mov Disord Clin Pract.* 2021;8: 420–426.

7. Arabia G, De Martino A, Moro E. Sex and gender differences in movement disorders: Parkinson's disease, essential tremor, dystonia and chorea. *Int Rev Neurobiol.* 2022;164:101–128.

8. Creeley CE, Denton LK. Use of prescribed psychotropics during pregnancy: A systematic review of pregnancy, neonatal, and childhood outcomes. *Brain Sci.* 2019;9(9):235.

37 An Irresistible Urge to Move

Sanskriti Sasikumar

A 36-year-old female presents to clinic with discomfort in her legs that has been causing her significant distress. Four years prior, she had received a diagnosis of restless leg syndrome (RLS) and was prescribed pramipexole 0.5 mg at nighttime. However, this discomfort has gotten much worse in recent months and is now occurring during the day, causing significant difficulty at her desk job. She describes her symptoms as "deep and aching" and at other times as if "ants are crawling" up her legs, and she paces around the room for some relief. Whereas previously her symptoms were exclusively nocturnal, they are now occurring in the late afternoon and early evening. She also has the same sensation in her forearms, although less frequently. She is otherwise healthy, with no other medical comorbidities. Her examination is unremarkable, with no lateralizing neurological deficits. Electromyography and nerve conduction studies are also normal. Blood work revealed normal ferritin and transferrin saturation levels. Pregnancy test was negative. A polysomnogram did not reveal periodic limb movements during sleep.

What do you do now?

RESTLESS LEGS SYNDROME

Restless leg syndrome is a sensorimotor disorder characterized by an irresistible urge to move the limbs that often occurs during periods of rest and relieves with activity. Its eponymous name is Willis–Ekbom disease, after it was first described by Sir Thomas Willis in 1672 and further detailed by Dr. Karl Ekbom in the mid-20th century. The symptoms can be challenging to describe, with descriptions ranging from a feeling of "restlessness, with an urge to move" to an "unpleasant sensation." Although it is commonly experienced in the legs, it can also occur in the arms, trunk, face, and genitals.[1] Symptoms usually occur at night, which can further interrupt sleep and quality of life.

Diagnostic criteria have been described by the International RLS Study Group (Table 37.1),[2] but the condition remains underdiagnosed despite being prevalent in the general population (9–22 cases per 1,000 person-years of follow-up).[1] The patient described in this case fulfills the criteria for RLS. However, essential considerations in the differential diagnosis include peripheral neuropathy, venous stasis, radiculopathy, drug-induced akathisia, and leg cramps.[1] RLS disproportionately affects women, with a 30–50% higher prevalence than in men.[3] This sex difference becomes apparent during late adolescence and is especially relevant during pregnancy, affecting one in five pregnant women.[3] As such, it is essential to test for pregnancy in women of childbearing age. Symptoms peak in the third trimester and resolve rapidly within 1 month after childbirth.[3] Recurrence can occur in up to 60% of subsequent pregnancies, and there is a fourfold increase in chronic RLS later in life.[3]

There is a bimodal distribution in the age of onset, peaking at the ages of 20 and 40 years.[1] However, diagnosis most commonly occurs in the fourth to sixth decades.[1] Periodic leg movements during sleep (PLMS), which can also accompany other sleep disorders, occurs in 80% of individuals with RLS.[2] A polysomnogram can be helpful in identifying these movements, as it can be challenging to obtain on history alone in the absence of a bed partner.

When assessing a patient with RLS, it is important to identify if it is primary (idiopathic) or secondary (symptomatic). Early onset disease (i.e., before age 40–45 years) tends to be associated with a positive family history (in 60% of individuals) and slowly progressive disease, in contrast to later-onset

TABLE 37.1 **Diagnostic Criteria for Restless Legs Syndrome, as Detailed by the International Restless Legs Syndrome Study Group in 2015**

Essential criteria (all must be met)	1. An urge to move the legs that is usually accompanied by, or felt to be caused by, uncomfortable and unpleasant sensations in the legs (or sometimes other body parts).
	2. The urge to move the legs and any accompanying unpleasant sensations begin or worsen during periods of rest or inactivity such as lying down or sitting.
	3. The urge to move the legs and any accompanying unpleasant sensations are partially or totally relieved by movement, such as walking or stretching, at least as long as the activity continues.
	4. The urge to move the legs and any accompanying unpleasant sensations during rest or inactivity only occur at night or are worse in the evening or night than during the day.
	5. The occurrence of the above features is not solely accounted for as symptoms primary to another medical or a behavioural condition (such as myalgia, venous stasis, leg oedema, arthritis, leg cramps, positional discomfort, or habitual foot tapping).
Supportive criteria (not essential for diagnosis)	1. Periodic limb movements (PLM): Presence of periodic leg movements in sleep (PLMS) or resting wakefulness (PLMW) at rates or intensity greater than expected for age or medical/medication status.
	2. Dopaminergic treatment response: Reduction in symptoms at least initially with dopaminergic treatment.
	3. Family history of restless legs syndrome (RLS) among first-degree relatives.
	4. Lack of profound daytime sleepiness.

Reproduced from Allen et al.[2]

disease, in which individuals are more likely to have comorbidities and increased RLS severity.[4] Genome-wide association studies have identified definite genetic risk variants.[1] Secondary RLS occurs with comorbid medical and neurological disease (Box 37.1).

Except in the context of iron deficiency, secondary RLS is similar in symptomatology and therapeutic response to idiopathic disease. In addition to serum ferritin, it is helpful to order transferrin saturation because

BOX 37.1 Comorbid Conditions That Occur With Restless Legs Syndrome

Major associations
   Renal failure (end-stage renal disease requiring hemodialysis)
   Iron deficiency
   Pregnancy
Other associations
   Drug/substance use
      Neuroleptics
      Histamine receptor antagonists
      Lithium
      Antiepileptics
      Antidepressants
      Antiemetics
      Alcohol
   Neurological disorders
      Polyneuropathy
      Migraine
      Amyotrophic lateral sclerosis
      Myelitis
      Syringomyelia
      Multiple sclerosis
      Spinocerebellar ataxia
      Myasthenia gravis
      Tourette syndrome
      Neurodegenerative disorders (e.g., Parkinson disease or multiple system atrophy)
      Rapid eye movement sleep behavior disorder
      Narcolepsy
   Rheumatological disorders
   Hypoxic conditions
      Chronic obstructive pulmonary disease
      Obstructive sleep apnea syndrome
      High-altitude/mountain sickness
      Sarcoidosis
      Pulmonary hypertension
      Lung transplant
   Cardiovascular disorders (e.g., hypertension)
   Obesity
   Diabetes mellitus

inflammatory states can mask low ferritin levels, as it did in this patient. This is especially relevant when previously stable symptoms worsen despite treatment. Iron replacement is the recommended treatment when serum ferritin is less than 75 μg/ml and transferrin saturation is less than 45%.[5] RLS symptoms manifest in 30% of individuals with iron deficiency, but the disorder has been attributed to a brain iron deficiency (due to abnormalities in brain iron acquisition) rather than systemic pathology.[1] It is important to recognize that medications can contribute to RLS symptoms—notably neuroleptics, antidepressants, and antihistamines—in which case the medication would have to be discontinued or the dose reduced. Therefore, obtaining an up-to-date medication history from patients is crucial.

When considering treatment strategies, it is helpful to classify the frequency of RLS symptoms *as intermittent* (symptoms occurring less than twice weekly), *chronic persistent* (occurring at least twice weekly), and *refractory* (unresponsive to first-line medications due to ineffectiveness or adverse effects).[6] This case describes an individual with refractory RLS. Nonpharmacological strategies are used for intermittent RLS in the form of regular physical exercise, avoidance of exacerbating factors (e.g., iron deficiency or white wine), acupuncture, pneumatic compression stockings, electrical or magnetic stimulation techniques, and cognitive–behavioral therapy.[6]

Dopamine agonists (pramipexole, ropinirole, and rotigotine) have been used as first-line therapy until recently. They work well to alleviate symptoms, with pulsatile dopamine agonists such as pramipexole and ropinirole providing rapid benefit with relief from 2 to 12 hours.[7] Rotigotine provides continuous dopaminergic stimulation and can improve symptoms that occur during the day and night.[7] However, these agents induce augmentation with long-term use, with one study identifying augmentation in 40–60% of individuals after 8 years of follow-up.[7] Augmentation refers to a worsening of symptom severity, which can manifest by earlier onset of symptoms compared to disease onset, increased symptom intensity, shorter latency of benefit from medications, and spread to other body parts. In the absence of other identifiable secondary causes, this is likely the case for the described patient, who was previously stabilized on pramipexole. Strategies to treat augmentation include reducing or splitting the dose, switching to a long-acting dopamine agonist, checking for aggravating factors (i.e., screening for secondary causes), or switching to an alternate therapy.[1]

Other first-line agents are $\alpha_2\delta$ ligands (gabapentin and pregabalin), the use of which avoids the risk of augmentation while providing the same clinical benefit.[7] These medications have the added benefit of improving sleep quality and can also treat comorbid anxiety or chronic pain. However, they do not improve PLMS. Rates of discontinuation due to adverse side effects were similar between dopamine agonists and $\alpha_2\delta$ ligands.[7] Opioids (low-dose methadone and oxycodone) can be considered as second- or third-line agents, especially for refractory RLS.[7] However, the benefit of these medications must be considered against the risk of opioid-induced respiratory depression and substance use disorder.

In this case, we opted to taper and discontinue pramipexole in favor of gabapentin. This bridging therapy worked well for the patient, with relief of symptoms on gabapentin 300 mg three times daily. She experienced mild dizziness when initially starting the medication, but this resolved over time.

Treating women during pregnancy is an important consideration, as current guidelines do not account for the teratogenicity of pharmacotherapy. Due to the limited safety data on $\alpha_2\delta$ ligands and dopamine agonists, they are not recommended in pregnancy. Instead, nonpharmacological strategies are first-line therapy. If symptoms are refractory to these measures, levodopa/carbidopa can be given in the evening.[8] However, the risk of augmentation must be considered, although the likelihood of occurrence is lowest in the third trimester.[3] Alternate options after the first trimester include clonazepam or oxycodone, dosed in the evening. During lactation, gabapentin can be safe because it is only minimally excreted into the breast milk.[8] Medication during pregnancy and lactation should be used at the lowest doses and for the shortest duration.

KEY POINTS TO REMEMBER

- Restless leg syndrome is a common disorder, with a 30–50% higher prevalence in women than men.
- Because management differs, it is important to categorize RLS as either idiopathic (primary) or symptomatic (secondary) and to rate the severity as intermittent, chronic persistent, or refractory.

- All RLS patients must be screened with serum ferritin, and iron supplementation is the treatment when serum ferritin is less than 70 µg/l and transferrin saturation is less than 45%.
- Dopamine agonists (pramipexole, ropinirole, and rotigotine) carry the risk of augmentation with long-term use, but $\alpha_2\delta$ ligands (gabapentin and pregabalin) can be used as first-line therapy because they have shown similar clinical efficacy.
- Treatment of RLS during pregnancy differs from the standard guidelines.

References

1. Mauro M, Garcia-Borreguero D, Schormair B, et al. Restless legs syndrome. *Nat Rev Dis Primers.* 2021;7(1):80.
2. Allen RP, Picchietti DL, Garcia-Borreguero D, et al; International Restless Legs Syndrome Study Group. Restless legs syndrome/Willis–Ekbom disease diagnostic criteria: Updated International Restless Legs Syndrome Study Group (IRLSSG) consensus criteria—History, rationale, description, and significance. *Sleep Med.* 2014;15(8):860–873.
3. Prosperetti C, Manconi M. Restless legs syndrome/Willis–Ekbom disease and pregnancy. *Sleep Med Clin.* 2015;10(3):323–329.
4. Rinaldi F, Galbiati A, Marelli S, et al. Defining the phenotype of restless legs syndrome/Willis–Ekbom disease (RLS/WED): A clinical and polysomnographic study. *J Neurol.* 2016;263:396–402.
5. Allen RP, Picchietti DL, Auerbach M, et al. Evidence-based and consensus clinical practice guidelines for the iron treatment of restless legs syndrome/Willis–Ekbom disease in adults and children: An IRLSSG task force report. *Sleep Med.* 2018;41:27–44.
6. Silber MH, Buchfuhrer MJ, Earley CJ, et al. The management of restless legs syndrome: An updated algorithm. *Mayo Clin Proceed.*2021;96(7):1921–1937.
7. Trenkwalder C, Allen R, Högl B, et al. Comorbidities, treatment, and pathophysiology in restless legs syndrome. *Lancet Neurol.* 2018;17(11):994–1005.
8. Picchietti DL, Hensley JG, Bainbridge JL, et al; International Restless Legs Syndrome Study Group (IRLSSG). Consensus clinical practice guidelines for the diagnosis and treatment of restless legs syndrome/Willis–Ekbom disease during pregnancy and lactation. *Sleep Med Rev.* 2015;22:64–77.

38 The Elderly Woman With Shaky Hands

Elizabeth Slow

A 65-year-old right-handed woman presents with a 5-year history of slowly progressive tremor of her hands. She notices the tremor when she is holding a glass of water or using utensils (especially when using a spoon to eat soup). Her handwriting has become messy and difficult to read at times. She likes to knit and play cards, and she finds that the tremor is starting to interfere with these activities. She has anxiety and is being treated with citalopram. She is otherwise healthy. Her father and paternal grandmother had a similar tremor. She has noted that if she has a glass of wine at dinner, her tremor improves. On exam, she has a slight vocal tremor. Her bilateral hands show tremor with posture and finger to nose testing but not at rest. Her neurological exam is otherwise normal. Vitals are normal. She recently underwent thyroid testing by her general practitioner, which indicated normal thyroid-stimulating hormone levels.

What do you do now?

Tremor is an involuntary, rhythmic, oscillatory movement of a limb around a joint. Tremor is further described by the position that brings out the movement (i.e., rest, postural, or kinetic), the part(s) of the body affected by the tremor, the frequency and amplitude of the tremor, and associated neurologic signs. These features can help determine the etiology of the tremor and therefore the most appropriate treatment. Some common tremor examples include a parkinsonian tremor—typically an asymmetric rest tremor—with a frequency of 4–6 Hz and associated with other parkinsonian signs (i.e., rigidity, bradykinesia, and postural instability). A cerebellar tremor tends to be a slow, 3–5 Hz, kinetic tremor that increases in amplitude as the hand approaches a target and is associated with other signs of ataxia. This chapter discusses common causes of symmetric postural and kinetic tremors, mainly essential tremor (ET).

ET is one of the most common movement disorders, affecting 1–5% of the population older than age 60 years, with increasing incidence with age. There are two peak ages of onset, in the second and sixth decades of life. A family history of essential tremor is very common (in up to 70% of patients), indicating a strong genetic component. Despite this, very few genes have been consistently linked to familial ET. Abnormal signaling in the cerebello-thalamo-cortical circuit is thought to underly the tremor in ET. There are no established neuropathologic criteria for the diagnosis of ET.[1]

ET is an action tremor—that is, it is evident when a patient performs an activity or during kinetic maneuvers in neurologic testing. The tremor in ET is brought out with posture holding—for example, holding arms extended from the body or during action maneuvers such as writing, drawing spirals, finger-to-nose testing, and pouring water from one cup to another. People with ET may have an action tremor in other parts of their body (e.g., head, voice, tongue, or legs). Bilateral arm tremor is required for the diagnosis of ET, with a duration of symptoms of at least 3 years. Supportive criteria for the diagnosis include improvement with alcohol and family history of similar tremor. The remainder of the neurologic exam should be normal. The somewhat controversial term "essential tremor plus" has been used for patients with the typical tremor of ET but other "soft" neurologic signs, including difficulties with tandem gait or a mild rest tremor

> **BOX 38.1** **Common Medications That Can Enhance Physiologic Tremor**
>
> Sympathomimetics (e.g., β-agonists for asthma)
> Amphetamines (e.g., cocaine and methylphenidate)
> Caffeine, theophylline, and nicotine
> l-Thyroxine
> Amiodarone
> Corticosteroids
> Lithium
> Valproic acid
> Selective serotonin reuptake inhibitors
> Tricyclic antidepressants
> Consider drug *withdrawal*: alcohol and benzodiazepines

as two examples.[2] The tremor in ET tends to worsen in amplitude over time and can become disabling for hobbies, handwriting/typing, and activities of daily living; hence, the previous term "benign" essential tremor is no longer used.

The main differential diagnosis for ET is enhanced physiologic tremor. Enhanced physiologic tremor can emerge in the setting of many different medications (Box 38.1), metabolic derangements such as hyperthyroidism or drug/toxin ingestion, or withdrawal (e.g., acute alcohol withdrawal). These factors can also exacerbate a previously established ET (or any type of tremor). In the setting of worsening ET, the above factors should be screened for and treated, if present. Physiologic tremor can resemble ET in many ways, including presence with action/posture, but physiologic tremor tends to be a higher frequency, lower amplitude tremor. Other differentials for ET include Parkinson disease (PD; but the tremor in PD is most often at rest) and cerebellar tremor. As mentioned previously, the tremor characteristics are often easily distinguishable from the tremor of ET. Dystonic head tremor is on the differential for isolated head tremor.[2]

Treatment of ET is symptomatic, with the goal of reducing the tremor amplitude to improve function. Exacerbating factors should be ruled out. Medications should be offered in the setting of functional disability or social embarrassment. First-line medications for tremor reduction include propranolol and primidone, with some studies suggesting up to 50% improvement in early, mild tremor. Topiramate can also be efficacious for the

TABLE 38.1 **Common Drugs Used to Treat Essential Tremor**

Drug	MOA	Maintenance Dose	Side Effects	Cautions
Propranolol Propranolol LA	Nonselective β-blocker	80–240 mg	Fatigue, bradycardia, hypotension	Asthma, diabetes (can mask hypoglycemia)
Primidone	Metabolized to phenobarbital; $GABA_A$ agonist + voltage-gated Na channels?	250–750 mg (start low: ¼ of 125 tab)	Acute toxic reaction, fatigue, ataxia, confusion, vertigo, nausea, unsteadiness	Elderly
Topiramate	Na, GABA,	50–400 mg	Appetite/ weight loss, paresthesias, concentration	Glaucoma, renal calculi

MOA, mechanism of action.

treatment of ET (Table 38.1). As tremor progresses over time, higher doses or combination therapies can be employed.[3] Patients may find tremor bothersome only in certain circumstances and use of low doses of propranolol on an as needed basis is sufficient. In severe, medication refractory cases, neurosurgical treatment is indicated through either deep brain stimulation or focused ultrasound.[3] Botulinum toxin has been trialed sometimes successfully for the treatment of ET but requires careful muscle targeting to avoid limb weakness.[4] There are new drugs in clinical trials for ET and wearables/assistive devices that may be of benefit in decreasing the tremor in mild/moderate ET.[5]

Most epidemiologic studies report no sex or gender differences in the prevalence of ET. Female gender is more closely associated with head tremor, whereas male patients tend to have a more severe postural hand tremor. There are no sex- or gender-related reports in differential response to treatment. However, care must be taken in the treatment of women with

ET who are planning to become or are pregnant. The common medications for treatment of ET—propranolol, primidone, and topiramate—are contraindicated in pregnancy due to possible teratogenicity. For this reason, most women prefer to stop taking medications during pregnancy. Drug diffusion to breast milk has been reported and low levels of topiramate have been found in breastfeeding infants, so care should also be taken during the breastfeeding period.[6]

KEY POINTS TO REMEMBER

- Differential diagnosis for ET is enhanced physiologic tremor, parkinsonian tremor, and cerebellar tremor. These can usually be distinguished based on the tremor characteristics, including position where the tremor emerges, body part(s) affected, frequency, amplitude, and associated neurologic signs.
- Physiologic causes should be screened for and ruled out in the case of worsening ET.
- Disabling/bothersome ET can be treated with medications, including propranolol, topiramate, and primidone, or surgery if severe.
- Caution is needed in treatment of ET for women who are planning pregnancy or are currently pregnant due to the teratogenic effects of common treatment medications. Caution in breastfeeding women is also indicated.

References

1. Welton T, Cardoso F, Carr JA, et al. Essential tremor. *Nat Rev Dis Primers*. 2021;7(1):83.
2. Bhatia KP, Bain P, Bajaj N, et al. Consensus statement of the classification of tremors: From the Task Force on Tremor of the International Parkinsonism and Movement Disorder Society. *Mov Disord*. 2018 Jan;33(1):75–87.
3. Ferreira JJ, Mestre TA, Lyons KE, et al. MDS evidence-based review of treatments for essential tremor. *Mov Disord*. 2019;34(7):950–958.
4. Liao YH, Hong CT, Huang TW. Botulinum toxin for essential tremor and hands tremor in the neurological diseases: A meta-analysis of randomized controlled trials. *Toxins*. 2022;14(3):203.

5. Castrillo-Fraile V, Peña EC, Gabriel Y Galán JMT, Delgado-López PD, Collazo C, Cubo E. Tremor control devices for essential tremor: A systematic literature review. *Tremor Other Hyperkinet Mov.* 2019;9.

6. Arabia G, De Martino A, Moro E. Sex and gender differences in movement disorders: Parkinson's disease, essential tremor, dystonia and chorea. *Int Rev Neurobiol.* 2022;164:101–128.

39 Chorea Gravidarum

Laura Armengou-Garcia and
Elizabeth Slow

A 31-year-old female presents to the family doctor for a 2-week history of new involuntary movements, with insidious onset, located in her face and right upper limb. She is a multigravida (G3P1) at 10 weeks gestation. She has a 3-year-old healthy son after an uneventful pregnancy. She had a spontaneous abortion during her first pregnancy 5 years ago and had a deep vein thrombosis 1 year ago. She takes a multivitamin complex and folic acid.

The movements do not interfere with her daily activities. Her husband remembers that she had similar movements during the first trimester of her second pregnancy.

Physical exam is normal except for a reddish blue to purple, net-like cyanotic pattern on the skin of both legs. Neurologic examination is normal except for intermittent choreiform movements of mild intensity in her face and right upper limb.

What do you do now?

Chorea gravidarum (CG) is a syndrome consisting of choreiform movements with onset during pregnancy. *Chorea* is the term to describe a type of hyperkinetic movement disorder that is involuntary, random, irregular, and purposeless.[1] The first report of CG was made in 1661 by Horstius.[2] At that time, its incidence was relatively high (1 per 2,275–3,500 pregnancies), and it was mostly related to rheumatic fever (up to 86% of the cases).[3,4] However, with the later widespread availability of penicillin, the incidence of CG dropped—to the point of currently being difficult to estimate due to its rarity.[3,4]

CG usually manifests in the first or second trimester of pregnancy and, in most cases, completely resolves during the third trimester or after delivery.[1] It may recur in subsequent pregnancies.[3,4] It can be unilateral or bilateral, and it usually involves the face and/or limbs.[4] It is present during the daytime and disappears during sleep.[4] Other symptoms that have been associated with CG include neuropsychiatric symptoms such as personality changes, depression, Tourette-like symptoms, hypnic hallucinations, delirium, and cognitive deficits.[3,4] Other case reports have demonstrated dystonia (an involuntary movement causing abnormal postures) as another possible hyperkinetic manifestation of the same syndrome.[5]

CG is a syndrome, and as such, it has different etiologies (Table 39.1). Traditionally, most cases were related to rheumatic fever in patients with a past medical history of rheumatic heart disease, recurrent tonsilitis, or Sydenham chorea in childhood/adolescence.[3] Acute rheumatic fever usually appears 2–4 weeks after a group A β-hemolytic *Streptococcus* pharyngitis. The most common manifestation includes acute febrile illness with joints and/or cardiac involvement. The less common form is the neurological presentation, also known as Sydenham chorea.[6] The differential diagnosis of CG also includes vascular causes (arteriovenous malformation, stroke, and central nervous system vasculitis), autoimmune disorders (antiphospholipid syndrome [APS] and lupus erythematosus [SLE]), endocrine disorders such as thyrotoxicosis or hyper-/hypoglycemia, Wilson disease, Huntington disease, neuroacanthocytosis (very rare), and drug consumption (cocaine, morphine, methadone, and amphetamine).[1,3] Finally, if all other etiologies are excluded, the diagnosis of idiopathic CG may be given.[4]

History and physical examination are key to working up the differential diagnosis and determining the underlying etiology (see Table 39.1).

TABLE 39.1 **Differential Diagnosis and Workup of Chorea Gravidarum Syndrome**

Cause	Clinical Clues	Investigations
Rheumatic fever (acute or recurrent)	Polyarthralgia, fever, carditis, subcutaneous nodules, erythema marginatum	ASO, throat cultures, ESR, CRP, echocardiogram
Vascular: arteriovenous malformations, stroke, CNS vasculitis[a]	Acute onset and lesions demonstrated in neuroimaging	Brain MRI
Autoimmune disorders: SLE, APS	Spontaneous abortions, arthralgias, DVT, dermatological manifestations	ANA, LA, aB2GPI, aCL, ESR
Endocrine disorders: thyrotoxicosis, hypo/hyperglycemia	Palpitations, fatigue, weight loss, heat intolerance, tremor, polyuria	TSH, T3, T4, thyroid ultrasounds, thyrotropin receptor antibodies, glycemia, HbA1c
Wilson disease	Neuropsychiatric symptoms, liver failure, hemolytic anemia	Serum ceruloplasmin, 24-hr urine copper, increased liver enzymes, genetic testing
Huntington's disease	Neuropsychiatric comorbidities, positive family history	Genetic testing
Neuroacanthocytosis	Parkinsonism, oro-lingual-facial dystonia, tics, social disinhibition, seizures	Acanthocytes in peripheral blood smear, brain MRI, EEG
Drug consumption: cocaine, morphine, methadone, amphetamine	Substance use disorder with behavioral, physical, and cognitive symptoms	Urine drug screening

[a]CNS vasculitis includes Behçet syndrome, Sjögren disease, immunoglobulin A vasculitis, polyarteritis nodosa, primary angiitis of the CNS, celiac disease, and sarcoidosis.
aB2GPI, anti-β_2 glycoprotein antibody I; aCL, anti-cardiolipin antibody; ANA, antinuclear antibody; APS, antiphospholipid syndrome; ASO, anti-streptolysin antibody; CNS, central nervous system; CRP, C-reactive protein; DVT, deep vein thrombosis; EEG, electroencephalogram; ESR, erythrocyte sedimentation rate; HbA1c, hemoglobin A1C; LA, lupus anticoagulant; MRI, magnetic resonance imaging; SLE, systemic lupus erythematosus: T3, triiodothyronine; T4, thyroxine; TSH, thyroid-stimulating hormone.

Spontaneous abortions, arthralgias, deep vein thrombosis, or dermatological manifestations from livedo reticularis to skin ulcers are highly suggestive of APS or SLE.[3,4] Blood work including complete blood count, anti-streptolysin antibody, autoimmune panel (e.g., antinuclear antibody, lupus anticoagulant (LA), anti-β_2 glycoprotein antibody I (aB2GPI), anticardiolipin antibody (aCL), erythrocyte sedimentation rate, and C-reactive protein, and thyroid function (thyroxine and thyroid-stimulating hormone) might be performed.[1,3,4] Throat cultures could be useful in patients with a history of streptococcal infections. If rheumatic fever is confirmed, an echocardiogram should be done to rule out possible cardiac complications.[4] Neuroimaging such as brain magnetic resonance, which is safe during pregnancy, could be done to look for structural or vascular causes.[4] If the initial workup is negative, Wilson disease could be excluded (with plasma ceruloplasmin and 24-hour urine copper testing), and Huntington's disease could be ruled out through genetic testing (especially if there is a family history of adult-onset movement disorders or psychiatric disorders).[4]

Different treatment strategies include targeting the underlying condition, the chorea itself, or the potential complications of the choreiform movements.[1] Symptomatic treatments for chorea are not usually needed because most cases are not disabling, and the movements tend to resolve upon delivery.[4] As a result, these treatments are exclusively for cases in which there is a risk associated for the patient or the fetus.[1] Complications of severe chorea include rhabdomyolysis, pain, hyperthermia, and weight loss. Chorea is usually treated with dopamine depleting agents such as vesicular monoamine transporter 2 inhibitors (tetrabenazine and deutetrabenazine) and dopamine receptors blocking agents such as neuroleptics (haloperidol and chlorpromazine).[1] However, both groups are generally contraindicated during the first trimester, when the risk of congenital malformations is highest.[3,4] Despite being classified as U.S. Food and Drug Administration category C during pregnancy, haloperidol and chlorpromazine have been shown to be safe during the second and third trimesters in low doses.[1] The American Academy of Pediatrics Committee on Drugs recommends haloperidol (0.5–2 mg twice or thrice daily) over chlorpromazine due to its lower anticholinergic, hypotensive, and antihistaminergic effects in the mother.[7]

CLINICAL CASE DISCUSSION

This patient had a clinical presentation in keeping with chorea gravidarum syndrome. She has a past medical history of spontaneous abortion, deep vein thrombosis, and examination revealed livedo reticularis on both legs. Blood work showed positive LA, aB2GPI, and aCL antibodies. She was diagnosed with APS and referred to hematology. She was treated with therapeutic dose of low-molecular-weight heparin and low dose of acetylsalicylic acid during the pregnancy. Because the choreiform movements were not severe, she was reassured, and no treatment was given. The movements resolved during the third trimester. After delivery, she was started on warfarin for the APS (which is contraindicated during pregnancy).[8]

KEY POINTS TO REMEMBER

- Chorea gravidarum is an infrequent syndrome that happens usually in the first and second trimesters and disappears after delivery.
- Investigations should be done to search for an underlying cause, and it should be treated accordingly.
- Treatments for chorea are reserved to the most severe cases and are usually given after the first trimester.

References

1. Miyasaki JM, AlDakheel A. Movement disorders in pregnancy. *Contin Lifelong Learn Neurol.* 2014;20(1):148–161. doi:10.1212/01.CON.0000443842.18063.a9
2. Cardoso F. Chorea gravidarum. *Arch Neurol.* 2002;59(5). doi:10.1001/archneur.59.5.868
3. Robottom BJ, Weiner WJ. Chorea gravidarum. *Handb Clin Neurol.* 2011;100:231–235. https://doi.org/10.1016/B978-0-444-52014-2.00015-X
4. Ba F, Miyasaki JM. Movement disorders in pregnancy. *Handb Clin Neurol.* 2020;172:219–239. https://doi.org/10.1016/B978-0-444-64240-0.00013-1
5. Donlon E, Moloney P, Frier D, et al. A case of new onset cervical dystonia in pregnancy. *Tremor Other Hyperkinet Mov.* 2022;12(1):33. doi:10.5334/tohm.734
6. Carapetis JR, Beaton A, Cunningham MW, et al. Acute rheumatic fever and rheumatic heart disease. *Nat Rev Dis Prim.* 2016;2(1):15084. doi:10.1038/nrdp.2015.84

7. American Academy of Pediatrics Committee on Drugs. Use of psychoactive medication during pregnancy and possible effects on the fetus and newborn. *Pediatrics*. 2000;105(4):880–887. doi:10.1542/peds.105.4.880

8. Alijotas-Reig J, Esteve-Valverde E, Anunciación-Llunell A, Marques-Soares J, Pardos-Gea J, Miró-Mur F. Pathogenesis, diagnosis and management of obstetric antiphospholipid syndrome: A comprehensive review. *J Clin Med*. 2022;11(3):675. doi:10.3390/jcm11030675

SECTION X

Cognitive and Behavioral Neurology

40 A Woman With Cognitive Concerns

M. Angela O'Neal and Sara C. LaHue

A 50-year-old woman whose mother has Alzheimer's disease (AD) is concerned about getting the disorder. She is healthy, without any significant medical problems. Her only medications are calcium and vitamin D. Her neurological examination, including a brief cognitive assessment, is normal. She asks about whether she should be on hormone replacement therapy.

What do you do now?

ALZHEIMER'S DISEASE

Incidence

The incidence of AD increases with age. The frequency of dementia doubles every 5 years beginning at age 60 years. The prevalence has increased such that one in nine people older than age 65 years has AD. AD disproportionately affects women. Women make up two-thirds of the caregivers for the disorder. In addition, AD is two or three times more common in women, which is not fully explained by women's longer life expectancy.

Role of Hormonal Replacement

Observational trials suggested that estrogen could play a role in delaying the onset of AD. However, the Women's Health Initiative Memory Study (WHIMS), published in 2003, demonstrated that estrogen, with or without medroxyprogesterone, substantially increased their risk of dementia of any cause, with AD being the most frequent etiology. This was a randomized controlled trial with two study arms, one involving 4,532 postmenopausal women older than age 65 years who received continuous combined estrogen plus medroxyprogesterone acetate or placebo and the other involving 2,947 hysterectomized women randomized to continuous unopposed combined estrogen or placebo. Overall, the risk of probable dementia for women in the estrogen plus progestin group was twice that of women in the placebo group, and the increased risk began to appear as early as 1 year after randomization.[1] A subsequent meta-analysis of 16 clinical trials (10,114 women) found that neither unopposed estrogen nor estrogen–progestin therapy protected against cognitive decline in older postmenopausal women.[2]

That the timing of menopausal hormone therapy (MHT) might be important was raised with an observational trial of 1,768 women followed from 1995 to 2006 in Cache County, Utah. The population-based study showed that women who used HT within 5 years of menopause had a 30% lower risk of AD, especially if the use of HT lasted longer than 10 years.[3] However, these observational results have not been supported in several recent large trials, including in an addition to WHIMS (WHIMS-Young) that demonstrated no significant benefit or harm to cognitive function when given to postmenopausal women aged 50–55 years.[4] An ancillary trial of the Kronos Early Estrogen Prevention Study (KEEPS), called KEEPS-Cog, found no cognitive benefit for women aged 45–54 years when using MHT up to 4 years versus placebo.[5] There is currently insufficient evidence to recommend use of MHT for the preservation of cognitive function.

Sex Differences in Alzheimer's Disease Risk

Some interesting findings may explain why women may be more susceptible to AD. It is known that the apolipoprotein E genotype with the APOE ε4 allele represents a major risk factor for AD. Farrer et al.[6] found that the risk of AD associated with a given genotype varies with sex. Women who had either the ε4/ε4 or the ε3/ε4 genotype were at higher risk to develop AD than men with the same genotype. Data from the Harvard Aging Brain Study show that women are more likely than men to accumulate amyloid and so have a larger amyloid burden when adjusted by age; subsequent studies have also shown elevated early tau deposition for women compared with men. There are also studies which suggest that earlier age at menopause may be associated with increased risk of dementia. This sex difference in AD is also seen in response to medication to treat symptoms, although evaluating potential sex or gender differences in response to AD medications is infrequently studied. For example, women with similar age, functional status, cognitive scores, and duration of AD show a more rapid cognitive decline than men treated with donepezil.

Prevention

As previously discussed, there is no role for MHT in AD prevention. However, many factors that increase the risk of cardiovascular disease, especially when present during midlife, are associated with higher risk of dementia. For example, midlife hypertension and obesity are associated with increased risk of dementia in later life.[7] Additional ways to address modifiable risk factors include regular exercise, smoking cessation, and participating in stimulating activities such as new learning and active socialization.

> **KEY POINTS TO REMEMBER**
>
> - Alzheimer's disease is two or three times more common in women than in men.
> - There is no role for hormone therapy in AD prevention or treatment.
> - Current best prevention of AD includes treatment of hypertension and diabetes, a regular exercise program, and engaging in activities that are both socially enriched and stimulating.

References

1. Shumaker SA, Legault C, Rapp SR, et al. Estrogen plus progestin and the incidence of dementia and mild cognitive impairment in postmenopausal women: The Women's Health Initiative Memory Study—A randomized controlled trial. *JAMA*. 2003;289(20):2651–2662. doi:10.1001/jama.289.20.2651

2. Lethaby A, Hogervorst E, Richards M, Yesufu A, Yaffe K. Hormone replacement therapy for cognitive function in postmenopausal women. *Cochrane Database Syst Rev*. 2008;2008(1):CD003122. doi:10.1002/14651858.CD003122.pub2

3. Shao H, Breitner JCS, Whitmer RA, et al. Hormone therapy and Alzheimer disease dementia: New findings from the Cache County Study. *Neurology*. 2012;79(18):1846–1852. doi:10.1212/WNL.0b013e318271f823

4. Espeland MA, Shumaker SA, Leng I, et al. Long-term effects on cognitive function of postmenopausal hormone therapy prescribed to women aged 50 to 55 years. *JAMA Intern Med*. 2013;173(15):1429–1436. doi:10.1001/jamainternmed.2013.7727

5. Gleason CE, Dowling NM, Wharton W, et al. Effects of hormone therapy on cognition and mood in recently postmenopausal women: Findings from the randomized, controlled KEEPS-Cognitive and Affective Study. *PLoS Med*. 2015;12(6):e1001833. doi:10.1371/journal.pmed.1001833

6. Farrer LA, Cupples LA, Haines JL, et al. Effects of age, sex, and ethnicity on the association between apolipoprotein E genotype and Alzheimer disease: A meta-analysis. APOE and Alzheimer Disease Meta Analysis Consortium. *JAMA*. 1997;278(16):1349–1356.

7. Gottesman RF, Albert MS, Alonso A, et al. Associations between midlife vascular risk factors and 25-year incident dementia in the Atherosclerosis Risk in Communities (ARIC) cohort. *JAMA Neurol*. 2017;74(10):1246–1254. doi:10.1001/jamaneurol.2017.1658

41 Memory Concerns in Middle Age

Sara C. LaHue and Marie Pasinski

A 48-year-old teacher confides, "I feel like my thinking isn't as sharp as it used to be. I never wake up feeling rested, and work is more stressful than it used to be. I'm worried I'm going to develop dementia like my mother." She has not made any errors at work, is the primary caregiver for her mother, and continues to manage her own family's household and finances without difficulty. She denies any other neurological symptoms.

Her recent history is notable for a 15-pound weight gain during the past year in the setting of perimenopause, poor sleep, and dysthymia. Her medical history is remarkable for prediabetes. She takes diphenhydramine to help her sleep. She drinks two or three glasses of wine per night. She does not exercise.

Physical exam is notable for blood pressure 148/90 mm Hg and body mass index (BMI) of 32.5. Her neurological exam is normal, including mental status and the Montreal Cognitive Assessment.

What do you do now?

MAINTAINING AND IMPROVING COGNITION THROUGH LIFESTYLE CHANGES

Memory concerns in middle age are common, typically benign, and can be improved by lifestyle modification. Although this patient performed well on cognitive testing, she has multiple risk factors for conditions that can affect her cognition, which if not treated may increase her risk of dementia in the long term.

Although some risk factors for dementia are not modifiable, such as genetics and advanced age, research suggests that lifestyle modifications can decrease one's risk of developing Alzheimer's disease (AD), the most common cause of dementia, and other forms of dementia, such as vascular dementia. Approximately 40% of dementia cases worldwide are thought to be attributable to the following 12 potentially modifiable risk factors: obesity, hypertension, diabetes, depression, physical inactivity, smoking, excessive alcohol consumption, hearing impairment, traumatic brain injury, lower levels of education, and exposure to air pollution.[1] Associated with these factors, sleep disorders are also a recognized risk factor for dementia. Some studies show that lifestyle interventions may improve cognitive performance. For example, the randomized controlled trial (RCT) Finnish Geriatric Intervention Study to Prevent Cognitive Impairment and Disability showed that a multidomain intervention of diet, exercise, cognitive training, and vascular risk monitoring significantly improved cognitive performance, including tests of executive function and memory.[2] There are several methodological challenges when testing how an intervention affects dementia risk, especially given the lengthy follow-up often required to identify the dementia outcome in a study population. Although this trial demonstrated short-term benefit, the long-term clinical impact of this multidomain intervention is less clear.

Steps to Optimize Brain Health

Assess General Health

Virtually every organ system supports brain function. Disturbances in pulmonary, cardiac, respiratory, hepatic, renal, immune, and endocrine functions can all secondarily impair cognitive function. Maximizing general health is crucial to achieving optimal brain health.

Hypertension, obesity, and diabetes, especially in midlife, are associated with increased risk of dementia in later life. Importantly, modifying these risk factors was shown to reduce rates of dementia. For example, the Systolic Blood Pressure Intervention Trial substudy Memory and Cognition in Decreased Hypertension, a multicenter study comparing intensive blood pressure (BP) lowering (target systolic BP <120 mm Hg) with standard BP target (systolic BP <140 mm Hg) was stopped early due to significant reduction in risk for major cardiovascular events in the intensive BP-lowering group.[3] Although the intervention showed a null effect on the primary endpoint of dementia, it did show a significant reduction in mild cognitive impairment (MCI) and a combined endpoint of MCI or probable dementia. Subsequent large meta-analyses have demonstrated that use of an antihypertensive medication in those with hypertension is associated with a reduced risk of developing dementia and AD compared to those not using an antihypertensive medication.[4] Cerebrovascular disease is associated with increased brain atrophy and increased white matter disease, but not amyloid deposition, and so the underlying mechanisms for the development of dementia may be distinct.

A common screen for cognitive concerns may include the following: complete blood count, a comprehensive metabolic profile, thyroid screening panel, vitamin B_{12}, folate, syphilis, HIV, and brain imaging.

Review Medications and Alcohol, and Tobacco Use

Be aware that medications, particularly those that are psychoactive and cross the blood–brain barrier, can impair memory and cognition. Chronic use of benzodiazepines and anticholinergics such as diphenhydramine (commonly used as sleeping aids, as in the case presented in this chapter) can affect cognition in the short term and have been associated with an increased risk of dementia in the long term. In addition, alcohol is toxic to neurons, and chronic use of excessive amounts is associated with reductions in hippocampal and cerebellar brain volumes, regions that are both implicated in dementia. For women, intake should be limited to no more than one standard alcoholic drink per day. Smoking is a significant risk factor for cerebrovascular disease and dementia, and its use should be discouraged.

Address Weight and Diet

Midlife obesity is an established risk factor for AD. Comorbidities including hypertension, decreased physical activity from osteoarthritis, and diabetes may be contributing factors. In addition, even in those who are not diabetic, insulin resistance may be important and negatively affect brain energy metabolism, amyloid clearance, and memory formation.

Many studies have investigated the contribution of diet, both macro- and micronutrients, on dementia risk. Numerous large observational studies support the "Mediterranean diet" as the best diet to decrease the risk of dementia and improve cognition, particularly the MIND diet (Mediterranean–DASH Intervention for Neurodegenerative Delay), which is a combination of the Mediterranean diet and the Dietary Approaches to Stop Hypertension (DASH) diet. The DASH diet, which is naturally low in sodium and high in potassium, has been shown to lower blood pressure. The DASH diet is rich in fruits, vegetables, whole grains, and low-fat dairy foods; includes meat, fish, poultry, nuts, and beans; and is limited in sugar-sweetened foods and beverages, red meat, and added fat. Studies have also shown an association between adherence to MIND and Mediterranean diets and less postmortem AD pathology on brain autopsy. Relatedly, higher daily consumption of ultra-processed foods was associated with cognitive decline over an 8-year follow-up period.

However, data from Mediterranean-type diet *interventions* are mixed. A post hoc subset analysis of the PREDIMED trial found that subjects in the Mediterranean diet group, compared with the control group, performed better on cognitive testing over a 4-year follow-up period. More recently, in an RCT of 604 cognitively normal older adults (BMI >25, consistently ate a suboptimal diet, and with family history of dementia), participants were assigned to follow the MIND diet or their usual diet, although both groups were instructed to also follow mild caloric restriction.[5] Antioxidant nutrient levels in blood were measured to support MIND diet adherence. Over 3 years, there was no statistical difference between groups in cognitive outcomes or brain imaging findings (e.g., change in white matter hyperintensities and hippocampal volumes). However, a Mediterranean-type diet has been demonstrated in RCTs to be associated with reduced risk of cardiovascular disease, including stroke, which may be associated with lower dementia risk long term.

Similarly, whereas nutritional deficiencies, such as vitamin B_{12} deficiency, can increase risk of dementia, the role of additional supplementation in the absence of deficiency is unclear. Furthermore, supplements can be a financial burden for patients, and in the United States, dietary supplements are not approved for safety or efficacy by a federal regulatory body.

There is currently insufficient evidence to conclude that a specific diet or dietary supplement will reduce the risk of dementia. However, patients should be counseled to limit processed foods.

Take a Sleep History and Treat Sleep Disorders

Certain sleep disorders are recognized risk factors for AD and are associated with the risk factors previously discussed, such as hypertension and obesity. Obstructive sleep apnea (OSA), the most common type of sleep-disordered breathing, is a recently recognized risk factor for AD and is treatable. In addition, irregular circadian rhythms increase the risk of MCI and dementia. This may be related to our growing understanding that neurogenesis and neuroplastic changes occur during sleep, as well as the chronic effects of hypoxia in OSA. Studies show that β-amyloid, which forms the amyloid plaques seen in AD, is cleared from the brain during sleep.

When proper sleep hygiene does not correct insomnia or fragmented sleep, consider a sleep study and referral to a sleep specialist.

Encourage Physical Activity

Exercise is one of the most potent ways to improve brain health, whereas physical inactivity is an important modifiable risk factor for AD. Although many large observational studies have found exercise to reduce dementia risk, the mechanisms underlying this association are likely complex and related to variables such as frequency and exercise type. For example, the benefit of physical activity may be synergistic by reducing the rates of other AD risk factors, such as hypertension, diabetes, and depression, and by improving sleep. Exercise is also associated with the increased release of brain-derived neurotrophic factor (BDNF), which promotes synaptic plasticity and neurogenesis, especially in the hippocampus. Numerous studies have shown that regular aerobic exercise increases brain volume on MRI volumetric brain imaging. Most notably, the size of the hippocampus, the center of memory and learning, becomes more robust when sedentary individuals engage in progressive aerobic training.

How this translates into real-world improvements in cognitive performance, however, is mixed. For example, a meta-analysis of 12 aerobic exercise RCTs lasting up to 26 weeks, and an RCT of a 24-month moderate-intensity physical activity program, failed to demonstrate differences in cognitive function between the intervention and control groups.[6] Interestingly, the cognitive benefits of exercise may be sex-specific, as one systematic review and meta-analysis found that women may derive greater benefit than men. Overall, there are numerous potential benefits from physical activity, and until more data are available on the effect of specific types of exercise, one should be encouraged to participate in the physical activities one most enjoys.

Screen for Depression and Anxiety and Offer Treatment

Depression across the lifespan is associated with an increased risk of developing dementia.[7] Complicating this association, however, is that depression which develops later in life may be part of the dementia prodrome rather than a risk factor for the disease itself. Similarly, a history of anxiety has been implicated in the risk for dementia and observed as a neuropsychiatric feature of the disease.

Although this association does not establish a cause, depression and anxiety are associated with increased levels of stress hormones and lower levels of BDNF—both of which have been shown to inhibit hippocampal neurogenesis.

Screening for these conditions and instituting proper treatment can improve quality of life and may, in turn, improve cognitive functioning. In addition, depressive cognitive disorders or "pseudodementia" may masquerade as dementia. In these cases, treatment of the depression reverses the cognitive dysfunction.

Promote Cognitive Stimulation and Social Engagement

Higher educational attainment and engagement in mentally challenging activities throughout life are associated with improved cognitive function and lower rates of dementia. Results from cognitive training trials have been mixed, and the most promising trials have been multidomain interventions rather than those isolated to cognitive training. For example, the Advanced Cognitive Training for Independent and Vital Elderly study found sustained improved performance in instrumental activities of daily living, but this program did not affect rates of incident dementia at 5-year follow-up.

However, there are still many benefits one can derive from engaging in cognitively stimulating activities. This is especially true for activities that also encourage social contact, which is a recently recognized protective factor and associated with reduced dementia risk. A systematic review of observational studies and low-quality RCTs found that older adults who engaged in social activities exhibited improved global cognition at follow-up. There is no physiological reason that we cannot continue to challenge our intellect with new experiences and new learning throughout our lives and reap the benefits of lifelong learning.

KEY POINTS TO REMEMBER

- Alzheimer's disease can be prevented or delayed.
- Up to 40% of cases of AD and other dementias are attributed to modifiable risk factors.
- Lifestyle interventions may be helpful in improving cognitive performance and decreasing the risk of dementia.

References

1. Livingston G, Huntley J, Sommerlad A, et al. Dementia prevention, intervention, and care: 2020 report of the Lancet Commission. *Lancet*. 2020;396(10248):413–446. doi:10.1016/S0140-6736(20)30367-6
2. Ngandu T, Lehtisalo J, Solomon A, et al. A 2 year multidomain intervention of diet, exercise, cognitive training, and vascular risk monitoring versus control to prevent cognitive decline in at-risk elderly people (FINGER): A

randomised controlled trial. *Lancet.* 2015;385(9984):2255–2263. doi:10.1016/S0140-6736(15)60461-5

3. SPRINT MIND Investigators for the SPRINT Research Group; Williamson JD, Pajewski NM, Auchus AP, et al. Effect of intensive vs standard blood pressure control on probable dementia: A randomized clinical trial. *JAMA.* 2019;321(6):553–561. doi:10.1001/jama.2018.21442

4. Ding J, Davis-Plourde KL, Sedaghat S, et al. Antihypertensive medications and risk for incident dementia and Alzheimer's disease: A meta-analysis of individual participant data from prospective cohort studies. *Lancet Neurol.* 2020;19(1):61–70. doi:10.1016/S1474-4422(19)30393-X

5. Barnes LL, Dhana K, Liu X, et al. Trial of the MIND diet for prevention of cognitive decline in older persons. *N Engl J Med.* 2023;389(7):602–611. doi:10.1056/NEJMoa2302368

6. Young J, Angevaren M, Rusted J, Tabet N. Aerobic exercise to improve cognitive function in older people without known cognitive impairment. *Cochrane Database Syst Rev.* 2015;2015(4):CD005381. doi:10.1002/14651858.CD005381.pub4

7. Elser H, Horváth-Puhó E, Gradus JL, et al. Association of early-, middle-, and late-life depression with incident dementia in a Danish cohort. *JAMA Neurol.* 2023;80(9):949–958. doi:10.1001/jamaneurol.2023.2309

SECTION XI

Pregnancy-Related and Peripartum-Related Conditions

42 Neurological Complications of Hypertensive Disorders of Pregnancy

Kristine Brown, Whitney Booker, and Eliza Miller

A 38-year-old G1 P0 patient at 36 weeks gestation presents with complaints of a new, severe headache. She has a history of migraines but has otherwise had an uncomplicated pregnancy. She describes the headache as severe, holocephalic, squeezing in nature, and worsened with activity. She says this feels different than her typical migraines, which are usually throbbing and unilateral. She has taken acetaminophen at home without relief. She also reports several instances of blurred vision over the past day. Upon evaluation, her blood pressure, previously normal, is 165/102 mm Hg. Her neurological exam is normal. Laboratory testing shows normal levels of hemoglobin, platelets, creatinine, and transaminases, as well as trace protein in her urine.

What do you do now?

PREECLAMPSIA

Clinical Features

The patient presented in the case scenario above has symptoms consistent with preeclampsia (PEC) with severe features. PEC is part of a spectrum of hypertensive disorders of pregnancy, which also includes gestational hypertension, preeclampsia with or without severe features, chronic hypertension with superimposed preeclampsia, HELLP (hemolysis, elevated liver enzymes, low platelets) syndrome, and eclampsia. PEC is defined as new-onset hypertension on two occasions at least 4 hours apart associated with evidence of organ dysfunction plus proteinuria at or beyond 20 weeks gestation.[1] Hypertension in pregnancy is defined as systolic blood pressure ≥140 mm Hg and/or a diastolic blood pressure ≥90 mm Hg. Proteinuria may be present but is not required for the diagnosis if other organs are affected. Eclampsia is defined as new-onset seizures in the absence of other causative conditions. The seizures may be tonic–clonic, focal, or multifocal. The diagnostic criteria for each hypertensive disorder are described in Table 42.1. PEC and its associated disorders are most common in the third trimester of pregnancy. However, new-onset PEC can also occur in the postpartum period. In addition to severe maternal morbidity and mortality, hypertensive disorders of pregnancy can also be associated with fetal complications, such as fetal growth restriction, preterm birth, and fetal demise.

TABLE 42.1 **Diagnostic Criteria for Hypertensive Disorders**

Disorder	Definition	Recommended Delivery Timing
Chronic hypertension	Hypertension diagnosed prior to pregnancy or before 20 weeks gestation	37–39 weeks
Gestational hypertension	New-onset hypertension (systolic ≥140 mm Hg and/or diastolic ≥90 mm Hg) at or beyond 20 weeks gestation in the absence of other symptoms, proteinuria, or lab abnormalities	37 weeks or at time of diagnosis if >37 weeks

TABLE 42.1 **Continued**

Disorder	Definition	Recommended Delivery Timing
Preeclampsia without severe features	New-onset hypertension at or beyond 20 weeks of gestation plus proteinuria (≥300 mg protein per 24-hr urine sample or urine protein:creatinine ratio ≥0.3)	37 weeks or at time of diagnosis if >37 weeks
Preeclampsia with severe features	New-onset hypertension in addition to one or more severe features, including severe hypertension (systolic ≥160 mm Hg and/or diastolic ≥110 mm Hg), lab abnormalities (platelets <100,000, creatinine >1.1 mg/dl, transaminases twice the upper limit of normal, or evidence of hemolysis), neurologic symptoms, and/or pulmonary edema. Proteinuria may or may not be present.	34 weeks or at time of diagnosis if >34 weeks
Chronic hypertension with superimposed preeclampsia	Chronic hypertension with progression to new proteinuria, rapidly worsening blood pressure control requiring increasing doses of antihypertensive medication, and/or other severe features of preeclampsia	34–37 weeks gestation based on the presence or absence of severe features
HELLP syndrome	Preeclampsia with associated hemolysis, elevated liver enzymes, and low platelets	34 weeks or at time of diagnosis if >34 weeks
Eclampsia	New-onset hypertension associated with seizure	At time of diagnosis regardless of gestational age

Pathophysiology

The precise pathophysiology of PEC is an ongoing area of research but is thought to be multifactorial, including uteroplacental ischemia, abnormal development of the spiral arteries, imbalance of angiogenic factors, endothelial cell dysfunction, and intravascular inflammation.[1,2] These changes combine to result in maternal hypertension and, in severe cases, multiorgan dysfunction. Renal impairment from preeclampsia is evidenced by proteinuria and often acute kidney injury; liver impairment is evidenced by elevated liver enzymes and, in rare cases, coagulation disorders; hematologic abnormalities are evidenced by thrombocytopenia and hemolysis; and neurologic impairment is evidenced by severe headache, visual disturbance, seizure, and/or stroke. Of note, headache and visual disturbance are common symptoms of PEC and must be distinguished from migraine, which is itself a risk factor for PEC.[3]

Treatment

Because hypertensive disorders of pregnancy are thought to arise from uteroplacental ischemia, the ultimate treatment is delivery in the case of antepartum diagnosis. The timing of delivery varies by disease severity and presentation (see Table 42.1). When PEC is diagnosed in the postpartum period, treatment is aimed at supportive care, treatment of hypertension, and seizure prevention. For patients with blood pressure ≥160/110 mm Hg, treatment with rapid-acting antihypertensives is recommended. Intravenous labetalol, hydralazine, and immediate-release oral nifedipine are the agents of choice in pregnancy. Intravenous magnesium sulfate reduces the risk of eclamptic seizures by approximately 50%, and it is recommended for patients with PEC with severe features, HELLP syndrome, and eclampsia.[4] Magnesium is administered as a 4- to 6-g bolus followed by 2 g/hr infusion through the time of delivery and 24 hours postpartum.

KEY POINTS TO REMEMBER

- Preeclampsia and eclampsia exist on a spectrum of hypertensive disorders of pregnancy.

- Preeclampsia can have new onset either before delivery or in the postpartum period. Headache and visual changes are common symptoms.
- Treatment involves delivery, rapid blood pressure control, and intravenous magnesium to prevent seizures.

References

1. Gestational hypertension and preeclampsia: ACOG Practice Bulletin, Number 222. *Obstet Gynecol.* 2020;135(6):e237–e260.
2. Jung E, Romero R, Yeo L, et al. The etiology of preeclampsia. *Am J Obstet Gynecol.* 2022;226(2S):S844–S866.
3. Adeney KL, Williams MA, Miller RS, Frederick IO, Sorensen TK, Luthy DA. Risk of preeclampsia in relation to maternal history of migraine headaches. *J Matern Fetal Neonatal Med.* 2005;18(3):167–172.
4. Altman D, Carroli G, Duley L, et al. Do women with pre-eclampsia, and their babies, benefit from magnesium sulphate? The Magpie Trial: A randomised placebo-controlled trial. *Lancet.* 2002;359(9321):1877–1890.

43 Third-Trimester Headache, Hypertension, and Seizure

Kristine Brown, Whitney Booker, and Eliza Miller

A 31-year-old G2 P1 woman at 39 weeks of pregnancy presents via emergency medical services after a witnessed tonic–clonic seizure. Her family reports that prior to the seizure, she appeared confused and complained of a severe headache. Upon initial evaluation, the patient appears drowsy but responsive to command. Her blood pressure is 152/99 mm Hg. Noncontrast head computed tomography (CT) is ordered for further evaluation. While awaiting her CT scan, she has a generalized seizure lasting 2 minutes. Magnesium sulfate infusion is initiated, and the patient is drowsy but otherwise stable. The decision is made to proceed with urgent imaging prior to transfer to the labor and delivery unit for delivery. Noncontrast head CT shows areas of hypoattenuation in the bilateral parietal lobes (Figure 43.1).

What do you do now?

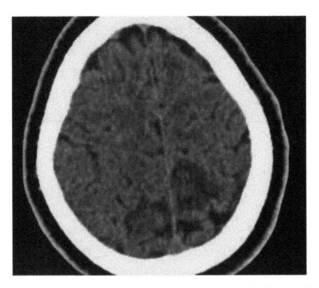

FIGURE 43.1 Noncontrast head CT shows areas of hypoattenuation in the bilateral parietal lobes.

POSTERIOR REVERSIBLE ENCEPHALOPATHY SYNDROME

Clinical Features

The patient in this case has the classic symptoms of eclampsia complicated by posterior reversible encephalopathy syndrome (PRES). PRES is characterized by vasogenic brain edema with resultant symptoms of headache and encephalopathy. PRES can affect all regions of the brain, although it is commonly seen in the parietal and occipital lobes. This leads to symptoms of headache (described as constant, moderate to severe in severity, and holocephalic), visual disturbance (including blurriness, scotomata, and/or cortical blindness), confusion (with progression to somnolence or coma in severe cases), and seizure. Symptoms are typically self-limited, and if present, visual disturbances usually resolve. However, in rare cases, PRES may be complicated by infarction or hemorrhage with associated persistent neurologic deficits.

Pathophysiology

Posterior reversible encephalopathy syndrome is thought to be precipitated by severe hypertension, endothelial dysfunction, increased vascular permeability, and disordered cerebral autoregulation.[1,2] This in turn leads to vasogenic cerebral edema and downstream symptoms. Changes may be seen in any region of the brain, although the parietal and occipital lobes are most commonly affected.[3] Untreated hypertension, including in obstetric patients with preeclampsia/eclampsia, is a well-established risk factor for PRES.[1] In fact, there is near complete overlap of the symptoms of PRES and eclampsia.

Treatment

Imaging is a key component of the evaluation and management of PRES. Although PRES is best appreciated on magnetic resonance imaging, noncontrast CT should be considered for rapid initial evaluation in patients presenting with severe symptoms due to the risk of intracerebral hemorrhage. Due to the high frequency of concurrent PRES in patients with eclampsia, rapid imaging should be considered in every patient with eclampsia. In addition to diagnostic imaging, the management of PRES is directed toward supportive measures to prevent and treat complications such as hemorrhage and herniation. Treatment of severe hypertension should be initiated (as described in Chapter 42). In obstetric patients with eclampsia or severe preeclampsia, treatment with magnesium sulfate is indicated for seizure prevention.

KEY POINTS TO REMEMBER

- Posterior reversible encephalopathy syndrome is characterized by vasogenic cerebral edema, and common symptoms include headache, visual disturbance, and confusion.
- Any region of the brain may be affected, but the parietal and occipital lobes are most commonly affected.
- Neuroimaging is recommended for all patients with PRES, including those presenting with eclampsia, due to the risk of hemorrhage and life-threatening cerebral edema.

References

1. Zambrano MD, Miller EC. Maternal stroke: An update. *Curr Atheroscler Rep.* 2019;21(9):33.
2. Miller EC. Preeclampsia and cerebrovascular disease. *Hypertension.* 2019;74(1):5–13.
3. Singhal AB. Posterior reversible encephalopathy syndrome and reversible cerebral vasoconstriction syndrome as syndromes of cerebrovascular dysregulation. *Continuum.* 2021;27(5):1301–1320.

44 A Woman With Severe Headache and Visual Disturbances Postpartum

Kristine Brown, Whitney Booker, and Eliza Miller

A 33-year-old G1 P1 patient who is postpartum day 5 after an uncomplicated vaginal delivery at term presents with complaints of a new-onset severe headache. She describes the headache as sudden in onset with intense pain from the moment symptoms began. She also reports blurred vision with spots in her vision that began at approximately the same time. She denies any medical history and reports her pregnancy was uncomplicated. Her vitals are notable for mild hypertension with blood pressure 143/92 mm Hg, and her neurologic exam is nonfocal.

What do you do now?

REVERSIBLE CEREBRAL VASOCONSTRICTION SYNDROME

Clinical Features

This patient has reversible cerebral vasoconstriction syndrome (RCVS). A sudden-onset, severe "thunderclap" headache that is maximal at onset is characteristic for RCVS. This may help differentiate RCVS from posterior reversible encephalopathy syndrome (PRES) because the headache in PRES tends to be more gradual in onset. Similarly, patients with a history of migraines will describe an RCVS headache as more sudden and severe than a typical migraine. Headache symptoms of RCVS may last for several hours at time of initial onset and recur over the following weeks. Other symptoms of RCVS include visual changes, such as blurring, scotomata, and, in severe cases, cortical blindness secondary to an occipital stroke or hemorrhage. Seizures and confusion are possible but less common than with PRES. In some cases, RCVS and PRES can occur simultaneously. Although RCVS is usually a self-limited condition, complications such as subarachnoid hemorrhage and ischemic or hemorrhagic stroke may occur. Due to vasospasm, ischemic strokes are often located in the watershed or end arterial territories. These complications can cause permanent disability.[1,2]

Pathophysiology

The pathophysiology of RCVS is not fully understood, but it is thought to arise from endothelial dysfunction, which leads to dysregulation of cerebral tone and transient cerebral vasospasm. Imaging in these patients typically shows multifocal areas of arterial vasospasm ("sausage on a string" appearance) that are usually limited to the intracranial vasculature. Of note, initial neuroimaging may be normal in up to 70% of patients with RCVS.[2]

Several precipitating factors have been associated with RCVS. RCVS was first described in postpartum patients, but it can also occur in nonpregnant patients of either sex. Multiple medications have been implicated as triggers for RCVS, including vasoactive agents (ergots, amphetamines, pseudoephedrine, phenylephrine, and epinephrine), immunosuppressants (cyclophosphamide and tacrolimus), serotonergic medications (serotonin reuptake inhibitors and triptans), and illicit drugs (cocaine, LSD, and Ecstasy).[2] When considering obstetric patients specifically, risk factors include preeclampsia or eclampsia and medications such as Methergine (used for bleeding/uterine atony) and bromocriptine (used for lactation suppression).[2,3] Other conditions associated with RCVS include migraine, pheochromocytoma, and systemic lupus erythematosus.[2]

Treatment

The treatment for RCVS is focused on accurate diagnosis (and exclusion of other acute diagnoses such as ruptured aneurysm), supportive care, and monitoring for complications (e.g., ischemic stroke and subarachnoid hemorrhage). All patients with RCVS (or acute thunderclap headache) should have neuroimaging and be considered for admission for monitoring and symptomatic support. No specific treatment strategy has been shown to hasten resolution of symptoms or definitively prevent complications. Prompt removal of a trigger, if one is identified, should be attempted if feasible. Close blood pressure monitoring is recommended. The severe headache symptoms may require treatment with nonsteroidal anti-inflammatory drugs (in nonpregnant patients) or even opioids. Calcium channel blockers are often used to treat headache and vasospasm. Triptans should be avoided because they may further precipitate vasospasm. If occurring in conjunction with preeclampsia or eclampsia, intravenous magnesium sulfate may be administered for seizure prevention. In cases of severe vasospasm causing ischemia, endovascular treatment with intraarterial verapamil may be needed.

KEY POINTS TO REMEMBER

- The most common symptom of RCVS is a thunderclap headache.
- The pathophysiology of RCVS overlaps with PRES, and both are commonly seen with preeclampsia or eclampsia in obstetric patients.
- Management involves neuroimaging, monitoring for and treating complications, and supportive treatment of headache.

References

1. Miller EC. Preeclampsia and cerebrovascular disease. *Hypertension*. 2019;74(1):5–13.
2. Singhal AB. Posterior reversible encephalopathy syndrome and reversible cerebral vasoconstriction syndrome as syndromes of cerebrovascular dysregulation. *Continuum.* 2021;27(5):1301–1320.
3. Kirschen GW, Hoyt K, Johnson E, Patel S. Eclampsia with RCVS: Postpartum seizure provoked by methergine. *Pregnancy Hypertens.* 2022;27:131–133.

45 A Woman in Labor With Hypotension and Dyspnea After Epidural Placement

Janet F. R. Waters and

Jonathan H. Waters

A 32-year-old female with history of significant obesity presented at 40 weeks gestation in labor. Blood pressure was 130/80 mm Hg, and pulse was 85 beats per minute. Epidural anesthesia was planned prior to vaginal delivery. Placement was challenging. A test dose of 3 ml of 1.5% lidocaine + epinephrine was given, immediately followed by 10 ml of 0.25% bupivacaine. Approximately 3 minutes later, the patient complained of inability to feel or move her legs. She then developed shortness of breath followed by marked hypotension, with systolic blood pressure of 60 mm Hg and heart rate of 40 beats per minute.

What do you do now?

EPIDURAL AND SPINAL ANESTHESIA

Total spinal block is a rare but serious complication of epidural anesthesia. It occurs when large doses of local anesthetic intended for the epidural space are inadvertently injected into the subarachnoid space.[5,6] This can produce anesthesia involving the entire spinal cord, nerve roots, and brainstem. When this occurs, patients develop weakness of the lower and sometimes upper extremities. Cranial nerve findings, including pupillary dilatation, may occur. Respiratory insufficiency ensues, followed by cardiovascular collapse with profound hypotension and bradycardia. Instant recognition and supportive treatment are needed to prevent maternal and fetal demise.[1] Patients may be placed in reverse Trendelenburg to prevent further caudal spread of the anesthetic agent. Intubation and positive pressure ventilation can be done to manage respiratory insufficiency. Hypotension may be managed with vasopressors such as epinephrine, norepinephrine, ephedrine, or phenylephrine. Bradycardia can be treated with atropine or glycopyrrolate. Urgent delivery by elective cesarean section may be indicated if fetal bradycardia ensues.

The primary factor that leads to a total spinal block is the failure to wait an adequate time following a test dose. A test dose is a small amount of local anesthetic with epinephrine, typically 3 ml of 1.5% lidocaine with 1:200,000 epinephrine. This test dose is intended to assess whether an epidural catheter has inadvertently been placed either in a vein or into the intrathecal space. If it has been placed into a vein, then the patient will experience tachycardia from the epinephrine and light-headedness from local anesthetic neurotoxicity. If the catheter is placed into the intrathecal space, the patient will develop lower-extremity paralysis; however, because of the small dose, the block does not spread beyond the umbilicus. Following a test dose, 3–5 minutes should pass prior to larger doses of local anesthetic. If this time is not given, then a total spinal block can result upon further dosing. Given full and immediate support, most patients with a total spinal block have complete recovery with no further sequelae.

Other Complications of Epidural and Spinal Anesthesia

Epidural Hematoma

Epidural hematoma occurs in 1 in 200,000 spinal anesthetics and 1 in 150,000 epidurals. Predisposing risk factors include spinal cord and nerve

TABLE 45.1 Anticoagulants and Waiting Period Prior to Neuraxial Procedure

Medication	Prior to Neuraxial Procedure
Fondipaparinux (Arixtra)	No recommendation offered
Clopidogrel (Plavix)	5–7 days
Abciximab (Reopro)	24–48 hr or until normal platelet function is demonstrated
Enoxaparin (Lovenox) high dose	24 hr
Enoxaparin (Lovenox) low dose	12 hr
Eptifibatide (Integrelin)	8 hr or when normal platelet function is demonstrated
Tirofiba (Aggrastat)	4–8 hr or when normal platelet function is demonstrated
Unfractionated heparin, high-dose intravenous continuous	4–6 hr and normal partial thromboplastin time
Unfractionated heparin, low dose	4–6 hr or after assessment of coagulation status

Source: American Society of Regional Anesthesia, Coags 2.9 (coagulation application for iPhone) (https://rapm.bmj.com/content/43/5/566).

root tumors, coagulopathy, and inherited and iatrogenic clotting dysfunction. Women with significantly decreased platelet counts due to HELLP (hemolysis, elevated liver enzymes, and low platelets) syndrome are at risk for this complication. Use of antiplatelet agents or anticoagulants can also sharply increase the risk of developing an epidural hematoma. Neuraxial anesthesia must be delayed until the effects of these drugs have subsided (Table 45.1).

Signs and symptoms of epidural hematoma include unusual back pain, numbness or weakness in the legs, and bowel and/or bladder dysfunction. Urgent magnetic resonance imaging (MRI) may be used to confirm the diagnosis. Emergency surgical decompression should be undertaken as soon as possible to reduce the risk of permanent injury. Diagnosis can be confounded by prolonged labor where a normal neurological exam is obscured by the presence of epidural anesthesia.

Spinal Cord Injury

Direct spinal cord injury can occur when neuraxial anesthesia is injected into the spinal cord instead of the epidural or subarachnoid space—in 80% of patients, the spinal cord and conus medullaris end at the level of the first lumbar vertebra, or L1, and in 20% of patients they end at the level of the second lumbar vertebra, or L2. Placement of the neuraxial block below the L2 level reduces the risk of injury. When this does not occur, direct injury to the spinal cord, conus medullaris, or nerve roots may occur. Patients will complain of pain or paresthesias in the lower extremities when a needle or catheter hits the spinal cord or conus.

Epidural Abscess

Epidural abscess is uncommon and occurs in 1 in 500,000 neuraxial blocks in the obstetrical population. Onset of symptoms may occur several days after the procedure. Skin flora are the most common infectious agents, with *Staphylococcus aureus* being the most common bacteria. Failure to adhere to aseptic conditions while placing a neuraxial block can increase risk of development. Prolonged use of epidural catheters beyond 3 days can also raise the incidence of epidural abscess. Immunocompromised patients are also at risk. Patients will present with fever, headache, back pain, leg weakness, and bowel and/or bladder dysfunction. Urgent MRI with gadolinium may confirm the diagnosis. Aggressive treatment with antibiotics is necessary. In cases of cord compression, surgical decompression may be necessary.

Meningitis

Meningeal infection is a rare complication of epidural and spinal anesthesia. It occurs in 1 in 39,000 cases. Microbial contamination from the mouth or the nose of the individual performing the block is the most frequent source. *Streptococcus viridans* is the most common agent. Use of face masks and sterile gloves reduces the risk of transmitting infectious agents. Clinical manifestations include headache, fever, neck pain and stiffness, and confusion. Seizures may also occur. Diagnosis is made by lumbar puncture, and treatment is with appropriate antimicrobial therapy.

Intravascular Injection of Local Anesthetic

This complication can occur during epidural anesthesia placement when a large amount of local agent is inadvertently injected into the vascular system.[7] Toxicity to cardiovascular and nervous system ensues. Bupivacaine is the most toxic, followed by ropivacaine, levobupivacaine, lidocaine, and chloroprocaine. Patients may complain of a metallic taste in the mouth, perioral paresthesias, double vision, and tinnitus. Agitation and confusion may occur, followed in some patients by seizures. Cardiac collapse may occur, with hypotension, arrhythmia, and cardiac arrest. Lipid emulsion is the treatment of choice.[8] A 20% intralipid should be given as a 1.5 ml/kg intravenous (IV) bolus over 60 seconds, followed by a 0.25 ml/kg IV (400 ml) infusion over 30–40 minutes. The infusion of lipid may be continued until cardiovascular status stabilizes. Continuation of cardiopulmonary resuscitation is necessary during lipid infusion. Some advocate for the use cardiopulmonary bypass if available. Recovery may take up to 2 hours. As discussed above, the use of a test dose is mandatory in order to avoid this complication.

Dural Puncture Headache

Dural puncture headache is the most common complication of obstetrical anesthesia.[2] It can occur after spinal or epidural anesthesia, which is typically used for elective cesarean section. It most commonly occurs when epidural anesthesia is administered for labor pain management and the dura is inadvertently punctured. The larger needle that is used for epidural placement allows greater cerebrospinal fluid (CSF) leakage than allowed by a smaller spinal needle.[3] Dural puncture headache results from this CSF leak through the punctured dura. This results in a low-pressure headache. Onset is usually within 24–48 hours of the procedure but can occur up to 5 days after delivery. Patients experience a diffuse headache upon standing, which improves within 15 minutes after lying flat. Traction on the meninges and meningeal vessels upon standing is believed to be the source of the postural symptoms. Some patients complain of neck stiffness or tinnitus with an echoing effect. Severe cases may result in cranial nerve six palsies with diplopia or tinnitus.

Treatment may be initiated with bed rest, caffeine, and hydration. If the symptoms do not improve after 24–48 hours of conservative management, then an epidural blood patch may be done by the anesthesiology team. This is performed by placing 15–20 ml of autologous blood into the epidural space.[4] The blood serves as a "patch" over the dural hole. The volume of blood may restore central nervous system pressure. Patients often experience immediate relief. Success rate is 70–97%. In some patients, a second patch is needed. In patients whose headaches are not postural, other possible diagnoses must be considered and appropriate workup initiated.

KEY POINTS TO REMEMBER

- Total spinal block may be prevented by ensuring that 3–5 minutes have passed after giving the test dose of local anesthetic and epinephrine prior to administering the full dose of the anesthetic agent.
- Administering neuraxial block below the L2 lumbar level reduces the risk of spinal cord and cauda equina injury.
- 22 headache is the most common neurological complication of neuraxial block. The hallmark is a headache that improves when the patient is supine. Persisting symptoms may be treated with an epidural blood patch.

References

1. Klein A. *Neurological Illness in Pregnancy.* Wiley Blackwell; 2016:70–79, 153–166.
2. Berger CW, Crosby ET, Grodecki W. North American survey of the management of dural puncture occurring during labour epidural analgesia. *Can J Anaesth.* 1998;45:110–114.
3. Turnbull DK. Shepherd DB. Post dural puncture headache: Pathogenesis, prevention and treatment. *Br J Anaesth.* 2003;91:718–729.
4. Crawford JS. Experiences with epidural blood patch. *Anaesthesia.* 1980;35:513–515.
5. Brooks H, May A. Neurologic complications following regional anesthesia in obstetrics. *Br J Anaesth CEPD Rev.* 2003;3:111–114.
6. Scott DB, Hibbard BM. Serious non-fatal complications associated with extradural block in obstetric practice. *Br J Anaesth.* 1990;64:537–541.
7. Dillane D. Finucane BT. Local anesthetic systemic toxicity. *Can J Anaesth.* 2010;57:368–380.
8. Brull SJ. Lipid emulsion for the treatment of local anesthetic toxicity: Patient safety implications. *Anesth Analg.* 2008;106:1337–1339.

46 Ringing in the Ears and Pain in the Head

M. Angela O'Neal, Janet F. R. Waters, and Jonathan H. Waters

A 26-year-old female is referred to you for evaluation of headache. The headache began 2 days after a vaginal delivery with epidural anesthesia, which required multiple attempts. She has a holocephalic headache, which is worse with sitting or standing and relieved with lying down. She also notes tinnitus, which is worse when sitting up. Her neurological exam is otherwise normal.

What do you do now?

LOW-PRESSURE HEADACHE

Pathophysiology

Low cerebrospinal fluid (CSF) volume is believed to cause sagging and traction on the nerves, particularly at the base of the brain. This sagging, when severe, can cause rupture of the bridging veins, leading to a subdural hematoma. Furthermore, sagging of the pons against the clivus may result in cranial nerve palsies. When there is loss of CSF, venous dilation occurs in order to maintain a constant intracranial volume. This pathophysiology explains the magnetic resonance imaging (MRI) findings in low-pressure headache: meningeal enhancement due to venous dilatation and brain sagging that may cause either a tonsillar herniation syndrome or a pseudo-Chiari malformation. The sagging of the brain may also cause apparent pituitary enlargement. A subdural hematoma can result from the stretching of the bridging veins. Following treatment, these abnormal MRI findings disappear.

Clinical Characteristics

The classic syndrome is a headache that gets worse in the upright position and disappears after a few minutes of being supine. The most common cause is a post dural puncture headache (PDPH), as in the case presented in this chapter. The headache is generally worse at the end of the day and is often, due to the continuity of the perilymph with CSF, associated with postural tinnitus. However, over time, the patient may not continue to have postural exacerbations. In addition, spontaneous low-pressure headache can occur where there may be no clear triggering event.

Evaluation

In a classic case such as the one presented, no further evaluation is needed. When the diagnosis is unclear, a brain MRI with gadolinium can be helpful in establishing the diagnosis. Although a lumbar puncture (LP) to check the opening pressure may be necessary, it is problematic because it is likely to worsen the headache syndrome.

Risk Factors

Low-pressure headache is much more common in younger individuals and rare after the age of 60 years. In the 20 to 30-year-old age group, low-pressure headache has been reported in up to 16% of individuals following LP. This is twice the reported incidence of individuals in the 30 to 40-year-old age range. PDPH is more common in women. Other risk factors include a low body mass index, a history of migraine, and a prior history of low-pressure headache. The risk of PDPH has been shown to be minimized by operator experience in minimizing trauma, appropriate orientation of the needle bevel, and using a smaller-gauge, non-cutting LP needle.[1] Figure 46.1 shows a number of different needle designs.

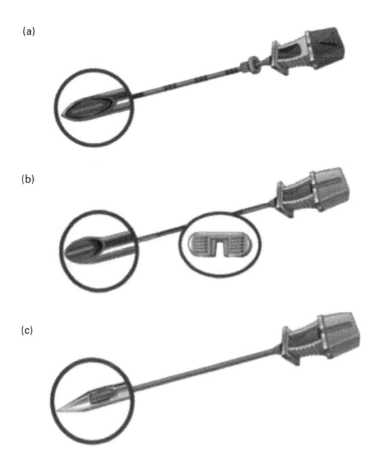

FIGURE 46.1 Three different needle tip designs. (A) The first needle is an 18-gauge "cutting" needle, which is typically found in a lumbar puncture kit. (B) The second needle is a 17-gauge Hustead needle, which is used for epidural catheter placement. (C) The third needle is a 25-gauge Whitacre needle, which is used for spinal anesthesia. Dural puncture headaches relate to the size of the needle and the type of point on the needle.

Treatment

The initial recommended treatment is bed rest with good hydration. Many patients' headaches will spontaneously improve with this alone. There has been some benefit shown from using caffeine in treating low-pressure headache. In a randomized controlled trial, 41 patients with refractory PDPH were given intravenous (IV) normal saline versus IV caffeine 500 mg. At 2 hours, the headache relief was 75% in the caffeine-treated group versus 15% in the normal saline group.[2] The use of oral caffeine 300 mg had marginal benefit in a placebo-controlled trial.[3] Multiple other agents have been tried that show modest benefit, including gabapentin, steroids, and theophylline.[4] Taking the patient's own blood and then injecting it into the epidural space—an epidural "blood patch"—is the gold standard of treatment. 90% of patients will have their headache alleviated after a single blood patch, and 96% after a second blood patch.[5]

Our patient was recommended to stay on bed rest for 24 hours and use acetaminophen and caffeine 1 tab every 4 hours as needed. If her headache persisted the following day, she would be offered a blood patch.

KEY POINTS TO REMEMBER

- Low-pressure headaches classically are alleviated after 5 minutes in the supine position.
- The findings on brain MRI reflect the pathophysiology and are related to brain sagging and the compensatory expansion of the venous system.
- An epidural blood patch is the most efficacious treatment.

References

1. Goadsby PJ, Boes C, Sudlow CL. Low CSF volume. *Practical Neurol.* 2002;2:192–197.
2. Jarvis AP, Greenawalt JW, Fagraeus L. Intravenous caffeine for postdural puncture headache. *Anesth Analg.* 1986;65:316–317.

3. Camann WR, Murray RS, Mushlin PS, Lambert DH. Effects of oral caffeine on postdural puncture headache: A double-blind, placebo-controlled trial. *Anesth Analg.* 1990;70(2):181–184.

4. Basurto OX, Martínez GL, Solà I, Bonfill CX. Drug therapy for treating post-dural puncture headache. *Cochrane Database Syst Rev.* 2011;(8):CD007887. doi:10.1002/14651858.CD007887.pub

5. Taivainen T, Pitkänen M, Tuominen M, et al. Efficacy of epidural blood patch for postdural puncture headache. *Acta Anaesthesiol Scand.* 1993;37(7):702–705.

Index

For the benefit of digital users, indexed terms that span two pages (e.g., 52–53) may, on occasion, appear on only one of those pages.

Tables, figures, and boxes are indicated by an italic *t*, *f*, and *b* following the paragraph number.

abatacept, 244
abciximab (Reopro), 317*t*
abortion, spontaneous, 165
absence seizures, 13–14, 15, 16, 17
absence status epilepticus, 16
acetaminophen
　for headache of IIH, 115
　for low-pressure headache, 324
　for migraine, 98, 127
　preeclampsia and, 301*b*
　for tension-type headache, 106
acetazolamide, 5, 114, 117
acetylcholine receptor antibodies, 151*b*,
　152, 156
acetylsalicylic acid (aspirin), 98, 238, 283
action tremor, 274–75. *See also* essential
　tremor
acute disseminated encephalomyelitis
　(ADEM), 66
acute inflammatory demyelinating
　polyneuropathy, 215
adenomas, pituitary, 120, 121
adrenal insufficiency, 121–22
adrenocorticotropic hormone, 121–22
Advanced Cognitive Training for Independent
　and Vital Elderly study, 297
aerobic exercise, brain health and, 295–96
alcohol
　brain health and, 291*b*, 293
　essential tremor and, 273*b*, 274–75
alemtuzumab (Lemtrada), 50*t*, 52*t*, 55
allopregnanolone, 4
a₂d ligands, 270, 271
Alzheimer's disease (AD), 287*b*
　hormonal replacement and, 288–89, 290

　incidence, 288
　prevention, 289, 290, 292–97
　sex differences in, 288, 289, 290
amantadine, 252*t*, 262, 263*t*
American Academy of Neurology, 187
American Academy of Pediatrics
　Committee on Drugs, 282
American College of Rheumatology, 242
American Congress of Obstetricians and
　Gynecologists, 84
American Heart Association, 84
aminoglycosides, 155*b*
amiodarone, 238
amitriptyline, 81*b*, 85*t*, 108
amphetamines, 41, 312–13
amyloid, 289, 295
anesthesia. *See also* neuraxial anesthesia
　genetic myopathies and, 163–64
　idiopathic intracranial hypertension and,
　116
angiotensin-converting enzyme inhibitors,
　161
angiotensin receptor blockers, 161
anisocoria, 129*b*
anterior pituitary, 121
anterior spinal artery syndrome, 181
anti-aquaporin-4 (AQP4) antibodies, 59*b*,
　60–62, 63
anti-B-cell therapy, 62–63
antibiotics. *See* antimicrobials
anticholinergics, 293
anticoagulation
　for cerebral venous thrombosis, 135–36
　waiting period prior to neuraxial
　procedure, 316–17, 317*t*

antidepressants, 26, 267–69
antiemetics, 115
antiepileptics. *See* antiseizure medications
antihistamines, 267–69
antihypertensive medication
   dementia risk and, 293
   ischemic optic neuropathy and, 237, 238
   for preeclampsia, 304
antimicrobials
   for epidural abscess, 318
   for meningitis, 318
   for neurologic manifestations of Lyme disease, 208, 211
   for post-treatment Lyme disease syndrome, 205*b*, 210–11
anti-NMDA receptor encephalitis, 71
   diagnostic criteria, 72–73
   malignancies and, 72, 74
   overview, 72, 74
   pregnancy and, 73–74
   treatment, 73
antiparkinsonian drugs, 251
antiphospholipid syndrome (APS), 279*b*, 280–82, 281*t*, 283
antiplatelet therapy
   epidural hematoma and, 316–17
   for giant cell arteritis, 244
   for Guillain–Barré syndrome, 214–15
   for ischemic optic neuropathy, 238
antipsychotics, 254*t*
antiretroviral therapy (ART), 185*b*, 186, 188, 190–91, 192
antiseizure medications (ASMs)
   bone health and, 7*b*, 8–9
   for catamenial epilepsy, 5
   cerebral venous thrombosis and, 135
   functional neurologic disorder and, 26
   for generalized-onset epilepsies, 12–13, 14, 15, 16, 17–20, 17*t*
   for migraine, 85*t*
   myasthenia gravis and, 155, 157
   polycystic ovarian syndrome and, 30

pregnancy and, 12–13, 15, 16, 17*t*, 18–20, 34–31, 40
   status epilepticus during pregnancy and, 40–41, 42
anti-Yo–associated PCD, 75*b*, 76–77
anxiety
   brain health and, 296
   in Huntington disease, 260, 263*t*
   in Parkinson's disease, 254, 254*t*
anxiolytics, 26
apolipoprotein E genotype, 289
apomorphine, 252*t*
aquaporin-4 (AQP4), 60, 61–62
area postrema syndrome, 59*b*, 60, 61
arrhythmia, 161
arterial vasospasm, 97
arteriovenous malformation (AVM)
   intracerebral hemorrhage and, 131–32
   overview, 130
   ruptured, 129*b*, 130*f*, 131*f*, 131, 132
   unruptured, 130, 132
arteritic ischemic optic neuropathy (AION), 236–38
arthritis, late Lyme disease, 207
arthrogryposis multiplex congenita, 156
assisted reproductive technology (ART), 35, 56
asymptomatic neurocognitive impairment (ANI), 187–88
asymptomatic neurosyphilis, 197
atenolol, 85*t*, 155*b*, 161
atrial fibrillation, 146
atropine, 316
attentional dysregulation, 25–26
aura, migraine with, 81*b*
   complicated migraine, 95*b*, 96–99
   defined, 83*b*
   diagnosis, 82, 83*b*
   stroke risk and, 82, 84, 87, 146
autoimmune disorders
   in differential diagnosis of CG, 280, 281*t*
   sex differences in, 208
autoimmune encephalitis, 71–74

Avonex, 49–52
Awater, C., 164–65
azathioprine
  for giant cell arteritis, 244
  for MOGAD, 67, 68
  myasthenia gravis and, 152–53, 153*t*,
    157
  in NMOSD management, 62–63

baclofen, 108
Bannwarth syndrome (radiculoneuritis),
    206, 207, 211
baricitinib, 244
B-cell-depleting agents, 48, 49, 55, 67
behavioral symptoms of Huntington
    disease, 260, 263, 263*t*
Bell palsy (BP), 207, 211
benserazide, 252*t*
benzodiazepines
  brain health and, 293
  for catamenial epilepsy, 5
  for generalized-onset epilepsies, 12–13,
    15
  for status epilepticus during pregnancy,
    40, 42
Bestaseron, 49–52
b-amyloid, 295
beta-blockers, 85*t*, 155*b*, 161. *See also*
    propranolol
bictegravir, 185*b*
biopsy, temporal artery, 243*f*, 243, 244, 245
birth. *See* delivery
bisphosphonate, 9
blood patch, epidural, 319–20, 324
blood pressure (BP), 293. *See also*
    eclampsia; hypertension; hypertensive
    disorders of pregnancy; preeclampsia
blood work
  for brain health optimization, 293
  for chorea gravidarum, 280–82
  for COVID-19 infection during
    pregnancy, 216
  for giant cell arteritis, 241*b*, 242

for status epilepticus during pregnancy,
    40
bone health, antiseizure medications and,
    7*b*, 8–9
bone mineral density scan (BMD), 9
Borrelia spirochete genus. *See* Lyme disease
botulinum toxin, 155*b*, 254*t*, 275–76
bradycardia, 316
brain-derived neurotrophic factor (BDNF),
    295–96
brain health optimization
  anxiety/depression screening, 296
  cognitive stimulation and social
    engagement, 297
  general health assessment, 292–93
  medications, alcohol, and tobacco use,
    293
  physical activity, 295–96
  sleep history and disorders, 295
  weight and diet, 294–95
brain MRI
  anti-NMDA receptor encephalitis, 72
  brain tumor during pregnancy, 221*b*,
    223*f*
  cerebral venous thrombosis, 134–35,
    135*f*
  Chiari malformations, 125*b*
  chorea gravidarum, 280–82
  cluster headaches, 102
  COVID-19 infection during pregnancy,
    216
  generalized-onset epilepsies, 12
  HIV-associated neurocognitive disorders,
    185*b*, 186, 187–88, 189–90
  Huntington disease, 261
  idiopathic intracranial hypertension,
    112*f*, 112, 113–14, 116
  ischemic stroke, 140–41, 141*f*
  low-pressure headache, 322, 324
  Lyme encephalitis, 207
  migrainous infarction, 96
  MOGAD, 66
  neurosyphilis, 197

brain MRI (*cont.*)
  optic neuritis, 229*b*, 230*f*, 230–31
  paraneoplastic cerebellar degeneration, 76
  pituitary apoplexy, 119*b*, 120*f*
  posterior reversible encephalopathy syndrome, 309
brain sagging in low-pressure headache, 322
brain tumor in pregnancy, 221*b*, 222–24, 223*f*
breastfeeding
  disease-modifying therapy and, 52*t*, 56
  essential tremor treatment and, 276–77
  Huntington disease management and, 262
  myasthenia gravis treatments and, 153*t*
  neuromyelitis optica spectrum disorders and, 63
  optic neuritis treatment and, 231–32
  by patients with multiple sclerosis, 49, 56, 57
  restless leg syndrome treatment and, 270
breech deliveries, 165
British Society for Rheumatology, 244
brivaracetam
  for generalized-onset epilepsies, 12–13, 17*t*, 18, 20
  pregnancy and, 40
  status epilepticus during pregnancy and, 40–41
bromocriptine, 122, 312–13
bupivacaine, 315*b*, 319
butalbital, 98

caffeine, 91, 98, 319–20, 324
calcitonin gene-related peptide (CGRP), 91
calcitonin gene-related peptide (CGRP) inhibitors, 86–87, 91, 98
calcium, 8, 9, 244
calcium channel blockers, 85*t*, 313
cancer
  anti-NMDA receptor encephalitis and, 72, 74

fertility preservation and treatments for, 221*b*, 222–24, 223*f*
  paraneoplastic cerebellar degeneration and, 76–77
  thymoma, 152
carbamazepine
  bone health and, 7*b*, 8
  for migraine, 85*t*
  oral contraceptive pills and, 34–35
  seizures and, 16, 17–18
  status epilepticus during pregnancy and, 40–41
  for trigeminal neuralgia, 103*t*, 108
carbidopa, 252*t*, 270
cardiac collapse, in intravascular injection of local anesthetic, 319
cardiac manifestations of Lyme disease, 207
cardiomyopathy, 159*b*, 160, 161
cardiovascular risk, migraine and, 97–98, 99
carpal tunnel syndrome (CTS), 169*b*
  anatomy and pathophysiology, 170
  clinical presentation, 171*f*, 171–72
  diagnosis, 172
  overview, 170, 173
  sensory loss in, 171*f*, 171–72
  signs and symptoms, 172*b*
  treatment and outcomes, 172–73
carvedilol, 161
CASCADE cohort (Concerted Action on Seroconversion to AIDS and Death in Europe), 188
catamenial epilepsy, 3*b*, 4–5
catechol-*O*-methyltransferase inhibitors, 252*t*
ceftriaxone, 205*b*, 208, 210–11
cenobamate, 8
Centers for Disease Control and Prevention (CDC), 198–99, 201, 202, 207
central core disease, 161, 163–64, 166
central nervous system (CNS)
  AQP4 in, 60
  COVID-19 infection and, 214–15

efficacy of ART in penetrating, 190–91
Lyme disease and, 206–7
cephalosporins, 208
cerebellar tremor, 274, 275, 277
cerebral angiography, 131*f*, 131
cerebral artery infarct, 214–15
cerebral blood flow, 97
cerebral hypoperfusion, 97, 98–99
cerebral vasospasm, 98–99
cerebral venous thrombosis (CVT), 133*b*
clinical features, 134–35, 135*f*
future pregnancies and, 135–36
incidence and pathophysiology, 134*f*, 134
overview, 136
treatment, 135
cerebrospinal fluid (CSF) diversion/ shunting, 115, 117
cerebrospinal fluid (CSF) leakage, 319
cerebrospinal fluid (CSF) loss, 322
cerebrospinal fluid (CSF)-specific effects of ART, 190–91
cerebrospinal fluid (CSF) testing
for anti-NMDA receptor encephalitis, 72
for HIV-associated neurocognitive disorders, 187–88
for idiopathic intracranial hypertension, 112, 113–14, 117
for optic neuritis, 230–31
for paraneoplastic cerebellar degeneration, 75*b*, 76
for status epilepticus during pregnancy, 40
for syphilis, 195*b*, 197, 198–200, 202
cerebrovascular disease, 293
cesarean section. *See also* delivery
COVID-19 infection during pregnancy and, 217
genetic myopathies and, 164, 165
for patients with generalized-onset epilepsies, 19
channelopathies, 160
CHARTER study, 191

chemotherapy, 222, 223–24
Chiari malformations, 125*b*, 126–27
childhood absence epilepsy (CAE), 12, 13*f*, 13, 15–16, 17*t*
children
congenitally affected DM1, 165–66
with MOGAD, 66
of women with MS, 57
chloroprocaine, 319
chlorpromazine, 282
cholinesterase inhibitors, 254*t*
chorea, 259*b*, 260, 262, 263, 263*t*, *See also* Huntington disease
chorea gravidarum (CG)
clinical case, 279*b*, 283
diagnosis, 280–82, 281*t*
overview, 280, 283
treatment, 282, 283
chronic hypertension, 302*t*
chronic Lyme (post-treatment Lyme disease syndrome), 205*b*, 209–11
chronic persistent restless leg syndrome, 269
citalopram, 254*t*, 263*t*
cladribine (Mavenclad), 50*t*, 52*t*, 54
clobazam
for catamenial epilepsy, 5
for generalized-onset epilepsies, 12–13, 15, 17*t*, 18
clonazepam, 39*b*
bone health and, 8
for REM sleep behavior disorder, 254*t*
for restless leg syndrome in pregnancy, 270
for trigeminal neuralgia, 108
clopidogrel (Plavix), 317*t*
clotting factor changes during pregnancy, 134*f*
clozapine, 254*t*
cluster headaches, 101*b*, 102–6, 103*t*, 108
CNS Penetration Effectiveness score, 190–91
cocaine, 41, 42, 280, 281*t*, 312–13

INDEX   331

cognition, lifestyle changes to improve. *See* brain health optimization

cognitive–behavioral therapy, 26, 87, 115, 269

cognitive impairments among PWH. *See* HIV-associated neurocognitive disorders

cognitive symptoms of Huntington disease, 260, 263

combined hormonal contraception (CHC). *See* hormonal contraception

complicated migraine, 95*b*, 96*b*, 96–99

computed tomography (CT)
arteriovenous malformation, 129*b*, 130*f*
brain tumor during pregnancy, 221*b*
complicated migraine, 97
COVID-19 infection during pregnancy, 216
ischemic stroke, 140–41
posterior reversible encephalopathy syndrome, 307*b*, 308*f*, 309
status epilepticus during pregnancy, 40

computed tomography (CT) angiography
COVID-19 infection during pregnancy, 216
giant cell arteritis, 242
ischemic stroke, 140–41

congenitally affected DM1 children, 165–66

congenital muscular dystrophies, 166

congenital myopathies (CMs), 160, 161, 164, 165, 166. *See also* genetic myopathies

congenital syphilis, 196, 200, 201

constipation, in Parkinson's disease, 250, 254, 254*t*

contraception, 34, 223–24. *See also* family planning; hormonal contraception

conus medullaris injury, 181, 318

conversion disorder. *See* functional neurologic disorder

cortical spreading depression (CSD), 97, 98–99

corticosteroids. *See* steroids

COVID-19 infection during pregnancy
clinical case, 213*b*, 217
diagnosis of neurological complications, 216
hypertensive disorder of pregnancy and, 215–16
increased risk of severe infection, 214–15
management of neurological complications, 216
overview, 217
risk of maternal and neonatal complications, 214, 216–17

C-reactive protein (CRP), 241*b*, 242, 244

cyclic progesterone lozenges, 5

cyclophosphamide, 73–74, 76–77, 244, 312–13

cyproheptadine, 85*t*

cytochrome P450 system, 8

dapsone, 244

deep brain stimulation, 251, 275–76

delivery
Chiari malformations and, 126–27
COVID-19 infection during pregnancy and, 216, 217
femoral neuropathy and, 175*b*, 176, 178
generalized-onset epilepsies and, 19
genetic myopathies and, 159*b*, 161–65, 167
hypertensive disorder of pregnancy and, 304
idiopathic intracranial hypertension and, 116, 117
lower extremity neuropathies associated with, 179–80
myasthenia gravis and, 156
for patients with generalized-onset epilepsies, 19
status epilepticus during pregnancy and, 40–41, 42
syphilis complications in, 201
total spinal block and, 316

dementia. *See also* Alzheimer's disease
  HIV-associated, 187, 188, 190
  lifestyle modifications in prevention of,
    292–97
  in Parkinson's disease, 254, 254t
depolarizing muscle-blocking agents,
  163–64
depression
  brain health and, 296
  in Huntington disease, 260, 263t
  in Parkinson's disease, 254, 254t
desflurane, 163–64
deutetrabenazine, 262, 263t, 282
diabetes
  brain health and, 293, 294
  ischemic optic neuropathy and, 237,
    238–39
  stroke risk and, 146
diabetes insipidus (DI), 121–22
diazepam, 40, 155
diet, brain health and, 294–95
Dietary Approaches to Stop Hypertension
  (DASH) diet, 294
dietary supplements, 295
diffusion tensor imaging, 189–90
dimethyl fumarate (Tecfidera), 50t, 52, 52t
diphenhydramine, 127, 291b, 293
diroximel fumarate (Vumerity), 50t, 52, 52t
disease-modifying therapy (DMT)
  breastfeeding and, 52t, 56, 57
  for multiple sclerosis in pregnancy, 47b,
    49–55, 50t, 52t, 57
distal weakness, genetic myopathies and,
  162–63
diuretics, 114, 161
donepezil, 254t, 289
dopamine, Parkinson's disease and, 250
dopamine agonists
  for motor symptoms of Parkinson's
    disease, 251, 252t
  for restless leg syndrome, 269, 270, 271
dopamine antagonists, 263t, 282
dopamine depleting agents, 282

dopamine transporter imaging scans, 251
Doppler ultrasound, 242
double vision, 75b, 151b, 319
doxycycline, 205b, 208, 211
D-penicillamine, 155b
drug consumption
  in differential diagnosis of CG, 280, 281t
  reversible cerebral vasoconstriction
    syndrome and, 312–13
  status epilepticus and, 41, 42
dual antiplatelet therapy, 214–15
Duchenne/Becker muscular dystrophy (D/
  BMD), 161
dural puncture headache, 319–20, 321b,
  322–23, 324
dysphagia, 162, 166
dystonia, 280
dystonic head tremor, 275

early disseminated Lyme disease, 206–7
early localized Lyme disease, 206, 207
early neurosyphilis, 197–98, 201–2
echocardiogram, 280–82
eclampsia, 304
  defined, 302
  diagnostic criteria, 302t
  myasthenia gravis and, 155, 157
  PRES and, 308–9
  reversible cerebral vasoconstriction
    syndrome and, 313
  status epilepticus and, 40, 41
  treatment, 304, 305
eculizumab, 62–63
efavirenz, 191
electrodiagnostic testing, 172, 176–78
electroencephalogram (EEG)
  anti-NMDA receptor encephalitis, 71,
    72
  functional neurologic disorder, 23b, 24
  generalized-onset epilepsies, 14f, 14, 15,
    16–17
  Lyme encephalitis, 207
electromyography, 176–78

INDEX   333

emtricitabine, 185*b*

encephalitis
anti-NMDA receptor, 71–74
Lyme, 207, 208

encephalopathy. *See* posterior reversible encephalopathy syndrome

endocrine dysfunction, 121–22, 280, 281*t*

enflurane, 163–64

enhanced physiologic tremor, 275*b*, 275, 277

enoxaparin (Lovenox), 317*t*

entacapone, 252*t*

entrainable tremor, 24

enzyme-inducing ASMs (EI-ASMs), 8, 9

ephedrine, 316

epidural abscess, 318

epidural anesthesia. *See* neuraxial anesthesia

epidural blood patch, 319–20, 324

epidural hematoma, 180–81, 181*b*, 316–17

epilepsy. *See also* antiseizure medications;
seizures
catamenial, 3*b*, 4–5
effects of treatment on bone health, 7*b*, 8–9
fall risk and, 8–9
family planning and, 29*b*–33*b*, 30, 33*b*
focal, 4–5, 29*b*, 30
versus functional neurologic disorder, 24, 25*t*
generalized-onset, 11*b*, 12–20, 13*f*, 14*f*, 17*t*
status epilepticus, 16, 19, 39*b*, 40–42

epilepsy with generalized-onset tonic–clonic seizures alone (EGTCS), 12, 13*f*, 16, 17*t*

epinephrine
reversible cerebral vasoconstriction syndrome and, 312–13
in test dose, 316, 320
total spinal block and, 315*b*, 316

episodic migraine prophylaxis, 91

eptifibatide (Integrelin), 317*t*

erectile dysfunction medications, 237

ergots, 98, 312–13

erythema migrans (EM) rash, 206, 208–9

erythrocyte sedimentation rate (ESR), 241*b*, 242, 244

eslicarbazepine, 8, 17–18

essential tremor (ET), 273*b*
diagnosis, 274–75, 277
overview, 274, 277
sex differences in, 276–77
treatment, 275–77, 276*t*

estrogen
Alzheimer's disease and, 288–89
brain tumors during pregnancy and, 223
in combined hormonal contraception, 82–83
migraine and, 91, 92
seizures and, 4, 30
stroke risk and, 82, 83–84, 87, 97–98, 146
trigeminal neuralgia treatment and, 108

ethosuximide, 15

European Alliance of Associations for Rheumatology, 244

Excedrin migraine tablets, 81*b*

exercise
brain health and, 295–96
for motor symptoms of Parkinson's disease, 251

eyelid myoclonia with absences (EMA), 12, 16–18, 17*t*

facial pain, 107–8. *See also* trigeminal neuralgia

facial palsy, Lyme disease, 206, 207, 208, 209, 211

fall risk
epilepsy and, 8–9
genetic myopathies and, 162–63

family planning. *See also* contraception;
hormonal contraception
cancer treatments and, 221*b*, 222–24, 223*f*

epilepsy and, 29*b*–33*b*, 30, 33
Huntington disease and, 261
Farrer, L.A., 289
fast-inactivation sodium channel agents,
16, 17–18
femoral neuropathy, 175*b*
anatomy and pathophysiology, 176
clinical presentation, 176–78, 177*f*
differential diagnosis of postpartum leg
weakness, 176–78, 178*b*
overview, 176, 181–82
retroperitoneal hematoma and, 178
sensory loss in, 176, 177*f*
treatment and outcome, 178
ferritin levels, 267–69
fertility. *See also* family planning
cancer treatments and, 221*b*, 222–24,
223*f*
epilepsy and, 30
fetal acetylcholine receptor inactivation
syndrome, 156
fetal outcomes
genetic myopathies and, 165
status epilepticus during pregnancy and,
40–41, 42
fibular (peroneal) neuropathy, 180
fingolimod (Gilenya), 48, 50*t*, 52*t*, 53–54
Finnish Geriatric Intervention Study to
Prevent Cognitive Impairment and
Disability, 292
fludrocortisone, 254*t*
fluorescein angiography, 231
fluorescent treponemal antibody absorption
(FTA-ABS) test, 195*b*, 199–200
fluoroquinolones, 155*b*
fluoxetine, 254*t*
focal epilepsy, 4–5, 29*b*, 30
focused ultrasound, 275–76
folate (folic acid) supplementation
idiopathic intracranial hypertension and,
114
for patients with epilepsy, 19–20,
34–36, 38

follicle-stimulating hormone, 30
fondipaparinux (Arixtra), 317*t*
Food and Drug Administration (FDA), 34
fracture risk, antiseizure medications and,
8–9
frovatriptan, 91
functional neurologic disorder (FND), 23*b*
evaluation and diagnosis, 24–25, 25*t*
overview, 24
risk factors and basis for, 25–26
treatment, 26
furosemide, 159*b*

gabapentin
for low-pressure headache, 324
for migraine prevention, 85*t*
for restless leg syndrome, 270, 271
status epilepticus during pregnancy and,
40–41
for trigeminal neuralgia, 108
galcanezumab, 106
general anesthesia. *See also* neuraxial
anesthesia
genetic myopathies and, 163–64
idiopathic intracranial hypertension and,
116
generalized-onset epilepsies (GEs), 11*b*
antiseizure medications for, 12–13, 14,
15, 16, 17–20, 17*t*
childhood and juvenile absence epilepsy,
15–16
epilepsy with generalized-onset tonic–
clonic seizures alone, 16
eyelid myoclonia with absences, 16–18
juvenile myoclonic epilepsy, 13*f*, 13–14,
14*f*
overview, 12–13
generalized tonic–clonic seizures (GTCs),
13–14, 16, 29*b*, 39*b*, 129*b*, 133*b*
general paresis, 198
genetic myopathies
impact on pregnancy and delivery, 159*b*,
161–67

INDEX   335

genetic myopathies (*cont.*)
 management of, 161
 neonatal outcomes, 165–66
 overview, 160
 types of, 160–61
genetic testing for Huntington disease, 261
gestational hypertension, 302*t*
giant cell arteritis (GCA), 236–37, 241*b*
 diagnosis, 242–43, 243*f*
 overview, 242, 245
 prognosis, 244–45
 temporal artery biopsy and, 243*f*, 243
 treatment, 244
glatiramer acetate (Copaxone), 50*t*, 52, 52*t*
glial fibrillary acidic protein astrocytopathy, 230–31
glioblastoma, 221*b*, 222–24, 223*f*
glioma, 223
glucocorticoids, 244–45. *See also* steroids
glycopyrrolate, 316
gonadotropin-releasing hormone (GnRH), 30
gonadotropin-releasing hormone agonists, 56. *See also* assisted reproductive technology
growth hormone, 121–22
Guillain–Barré syndrome (GBS), 214–15

haloperidol, 71, 282
Harvard Aging Brain Study, 289
headache diary, 86, 90–91
headache disorders. *See also* migraine
 arteriovenous malformation, 129*b*, 130*f*, 130–32
 cerebral venous thrombosis, 133*b*, 134*f*, 134–36, 135*f*
 Chiari malformations, 125*b*, 126–27
 dural puncture headache, 319–20
 idiopathic intracranial hypertension, 111*b*, 112*f*, 112–17, 113*b*
 low-pressure headache, 321*b*, 322–24, 323*f*
 pituitary apoplexy, 119*b*, 120*f*, 120–22

posterior reversible encephalopathy syndrome, 307*b*, 308
 in preeclampsia, 301*b*, 304
 primary, 101*b*, 102–8, 103*t*, 105*b*, 107*b*
 reversible cerebral vasoconstriction syndrome, 311*b*, 312, 313
"Headache in Pregnancy and Lactation" (Rayhill), 87
heart failure, 161
HELLP (hemolysis, elevated liver enzymes, low platelets) syndrome, 302, 302*t*, 304, 316–17
hematologic abnormalities from preeclampsia, 304
hemicrania continua, 103*t*
hemorrhage
 intracerebral, 129*b*, 130*f*, 130, 131–32
 postpartum, 165
hemorrhagic stroke, 83–84
heparin
 for antiphospholipid syndrome, 283
 for cerebral venous thrombosis, 135–36
 waiting period prior to neuraxial procedure, 317*t*
hereditary myopathies. *See* genetic myopathies
herpes simplex virus (HSV), 71, 72
highly active antiretroviral therapy (HAART), 190, 191
HIV-associated dementia (HAD), 187, 188, 190
HIV-associated neurocognitive disorders (HAND), 185*b*
 changing epidemiology of HIV and, 186–87
 classification and presentation, 187–88
 comorbidity management and, 189, 191, 192
 diagnosis, 189–90
 overview, 186, 192
 pathogenesis, epidemiology, and predictors of, 188

prognosis and response to treatment, 190–91
sex differences in, 186–87, 189
HIV Dementia Scale, 185b, 189
Hoover sign, 24
hormonal contraception, 34
    antiseizure medications and, 34–35
    brain tumors during pregnancy and, 223
    for catamenial epilepsy, 5
    interactions with migraine medications, 85–86, 85t
    migraine and, 81b, 82–86, 85t, 87, 92
    progesterone-only, 86, 97–98
    stroke risk and, 82, 83–84, 87, 97–98, 146
    trigeminal neuralgia treatment and, 108
hormonal therapy
    Alzheimer's disease and, 288–89, 290
    brain tumors during pregnancy and, 223
    for migraine, 92
    stroke risk and, 146
    trigeminal neuralgia treatment and, 108
hormones
    autoimmune disease and, 208
    brain tumors during pregnancy and, 223
    Parkinson's disease medications and, 251, 257
    pituitary apoplexy and, 121–22
    seizures and, 30
Horton disease. See giant cell arteritis
Humphrey visual field testing, 114, 115
Huntington disease (HD), 259b
    cognitive symptoms, 260, 263
    diagnosis, 261
    in differential diagnosis of CG, 280–82, 281t
    genetics of, 260–61
    management of, 261–62, 263t
    motor symptoms, 259b, 260, 263, 263t
    overview, 260, 263
    patient resources, 261, 262t
    psychiatric/behavioral symptoms, 260, 263, 263t
    sex differences in, 261

hydralazine, 304
hydrocortisone, 122
hypercapnia, 162
hypercoagulability workup, 135
hypertension. See also hypertensive disorders of pregnancy
    brain health and, 293
    chronic, 302t
    COVID-19 infection during pregnancy and, 214
    idiopathic intracranial, 111b, 112f, 112–17, 113b
    ischemic optic neuropathy and, 237, 238
    in pregnancy, 302
    PRES and, 308–9
    stroke risk and, 146
hypertensive disorders of pregnancy (HDP). See also eclampsia; preeclampsia
    clinical features, 302
    COVID-19 infection and, 215–16, 217
    diagnostic criteria, 302, 302t
    overview, 304–5
    treatment, 304
hyperventilation, 14, 15
hypogonadotropic deficiency, 121–22
hypotension after epidural placement, 315b, 316
hypothalamic dysfunction, 30
hypothyroidism, 121–22
hypoxemia, 162

ibuprofen, 115
idiopathic intracranial hypertension (IIH), 111b
    diagnostic criteria, 113b
    management during labor and birth, 116
    overview, 112f, 112–14, 116–17
    treatment, 114–15
IIH Life study, 116
immediate-release oral nifedipine, 304
immune response, sex differences in, 208–9

INDEX   337

immunoglobulins
  for anti-NMDA receptor encephalitis, 73–74
  COVID-19 infection during pregnancy and, 214–15
  for MOGAD, 67, 68
  for MS relapse during pregnancy, 49
  for myasthenia gravis, 152–53, 153*t*, 156, 157
  for optic neuritis, 231–32, 236
  for paraneoplastic cerebellar degeneration, 76–77
  for post-treatment Lyme disease syndrome, 205*b*, 210–11
immunosuppression. *See also* azathioprine
  for anti-NMDA receptor encephalitis, 73–74
  for MOGAD, 67, 68
  in NMOSD management, 62–63
  reversible cerebral vasoconstriction syndrome and, 312–13
inadequate luteal pattern (C3), catamenial epilepsy, 4, 5
indomethacin, 103*t*
inebilizumab, 62–63
Infectious Diseases Society of America (IDSA), 210–11
infertility, cancer treatment-related, 222
inhalation anesthetics, 163–64
inherited myopathies. *See* genetic myopathies
insulin resistance, 294
intensive blood pressure (BP) lowering, 293
interferons, 49–52, 50*t*, 52*t*, 238
intermittent restless leg syndrome, 269
International Classification of Headache Disorders, third edition (ICHD-3), 82, 90, 96*b*, 96, 113*b*
International Headache Society, 84
International Restless Legs Syndrome Study Group, 266, 267*t*
intracerebral hemorrhage (ICH), 129*b*, 130*f*, 130, 131–32

intracranial pressure (ICP). *See also* idiopathic intracranial hypertension
  cerebral venous thrombosis and, 134–35
  Chiari malformations and, 126
intrapartum syphilis, 196, 200–1
intravascular injection of local anesthetic, 319
intravenous (IV) thrombolysis, 141
intravenous immunoglobulin (IVIG)
  for anti-NMDA receptor encephalitis, 73–74
  COVID-19 infection during pregnancy and, 214–15
  for MOGAD, 67, 68
  for MS relapse during pregnancy, 49
  for myasthenia gravis, 152–53, 156, 157
  for optic neuritis, 231–32, 236
  for paraneoplastic cerebellar degeneration, 76–77
  for post-treatment Lyme disease syndrome, 205*b*, 210–11
inverse agonist/antagonist serotonin 5-HT, 254*t*
iodinated contrast agents, 155*b*
iron deficiency, 267–69, 271
ischemic optic neuropathy (ION), 235*b*, 236*f*
  diagnosis, 237
  distinguishing between nonvasculitic and vasculitic, 237–38
  overview, 236–37
  treatment and prognosis, 238–39
ischemic stroke (IS)
  incidence and etiology, 140
  migraine and, 84, 97, 98
  migrainous infarction, 95*b*, 96*b*, 96–97
  oral contraceptive pills and, 83–84
  in pregnancy, 139*b*, 140–42, 141*f*, 142*f*
  reversible cerebral vasoconstriction syndrome and, 312
  treatment, 140–41
isoflurane, 163–64
Ixodes ticks, 206. *See also* Lyme disease

Jeavons syndrome. *See* eyelid myoclonia with absences
juvenile absence epilepsy (JAE), 12, 13*f*, 16, 17*t*
juvenile myoclonic epilepsy (JME), 13*f*, 14*f*
  antiseizure medications for, 14, 17*t*, 18–20
  clinical case, 11*b*
  overview, 12, 13–14
juvenile-onset Huntington disease, 260–61

ketamine, 40–41
kinetic tremor, 274. *See also* essential tremor
Kronos Early Estrogen Prevention Study (KEEPS)-Cog, 288–89
kyphoscoliosis, 162, 164

labetalol, 304
labor. *See* delivery
lacosamide
  for generalized-onset epilepsies, 12–13, 17*t*, 18
  pregnancy and, 40
  status epilepticus during pregnancy and, 40–41
lactation. *See* breastfeeding
lamotrigine
  bone health and, 8
  for generalized-onset epilepsies, 12–13, 14, 15, 16, 17*t*, 18, 19–20
  oral contraceptive pills and, 34–35
  polycystic ovarian syndrome and, 30, 33*b*
  pregnancy and, 34, 36*b*–37, 36
  seizures and, 17–18
  status epilepticus during pregnancy and, 40–41
  for trigeminal autonomic cephalgiasa, 103*t*
  for trigeminal neuralgia, 108
large-vessel occlusion, 214–15
late Lyme disease, 207
late neurosyphilis, 197, 198, 201–2
latent phase of syphilis, 196–97

lateral femoral cutaneous neuropathy (meralgia paresthetica), 179–80
leflunomide, 244
leg weakness, postpartum. *See* postpartum leg weakness
levetiracetam, 39*b*
  bone health and, 8
  for generalized-onset epilepsies, 12–13, 14, 15, 16, 17*t*, 18, 19–20
  myasthenia gravis and, 155, 157
  polycystic ovarian syndrome and, 30
  pregnancy and, 34, 36, 40
  seizures and, 3*b*, 17–18
levobupivacaine, 319
levodopa
  for motor symptoms of Parkinson's disease, 251, 252*t*
  pregnancy and, 251
  for restless leg syndrome in pregnancy, 270
Lewy bodies, 250
lidocaine, 315*b*, 316, 319
"Life's Essential 8", 146
lifestyle changes
  brain health optimization through, 292–97
  for headache of IIH, 115
limb–girdle muscular dystrophy (LGMD) type 2D, 159*b*, 164–65
lipid infusion, 319
lithium, 106
liver impairment from preeclampsia, 304
local anesthetic
  intravascular injection of, 319
  in test dose, 316, 320
  total spinal block and, 315*b*, 316
lower extremity neuropathies associated with pregnancy and delivery, 179–80. *See also* femoral neuropathy
low-pressure headache, 321*b*
  clinical characteristics, 322
  evaluation, 322
  pathophysiology, 322, 324

low-pressure headache (*cont.*)
  risk factors, 322–23, 323*f*
  treatment, 324
LSD, 312–13
lumbar puncture (LP)
  for idiopathic intracranial hypertension,
    112–13, 115, 117
  low-pressure headache and, 322–23
  for meningitis, 318
  needle tip designs for, 323*f*
  for syphilis, 195*b*, 198–200, 202
lumbosacral plexus neuropathy, 180
lung function, genetic myopathies and, 164
lupus erythematosus, 280–82, 281*t*,
    312–13
luteal phase, 4
luteinizing hormone, 30
Lyme disease
  clinical manifestations, 206–7
  overview, 211
  pathogenesis and epidemiology, 206
  post-treatment Lyme disease syndrome,
    205*b*, 209–11
  sex and gender differences in, 208–9
  sociocultural differences and, 209
  treatment, 208
Lyme disease facial palsy (LDFP), 206, 207,
    208, 209, 211
Lyme encephalitis, 207, 208
Lyme neuroborreliosis, 207, 208–9
lymphocytic meningitis, 206–7

macrolide antibiotics, 155*b*
magnesium
  for headache of IIH, 115
  for hypertensive disorders of pregnancy,
    304, 305
  for migraine prophylaxis, 91
  myasthenia gravis and, 155*b*, 155, 157
  pregnancy and, 40
  for PRES, 307*b*, 309
  for reversible cerebral vasoconstriction
    syndrome, 313

magnetic resonance angiography (MRA)
  ischemic stroke, 140–41, 142*f*
  meningovascular syphilis, 197–98
  status epilepticus during pregnancy, 40
magnetic resonance arteriogram, 134–35,
    135*f*
magnetic resonance imaging (MRI). *See also*
    brain MRI
  anterior spinal artery syndrome, 181
  epidural abscess, 318
  epidural hematoma, 180–81, 317
  status epilepticus during pregnancy, 40
magnetic resonance spectroscopy (MRS),
    189–90
magnetic resonance venogram (MRV),
    125*b*
  cerebral venous thrombosis, 134–35,
    135*f*
  idiopathic intracranial hypertension, 112
major congenital malformations (MCMs),
    34
malignancies
  anti-NMDA receptor encephalitis and,
    72, 74
  fertility preservation and treatments for,
    221*b*, 222–24, 223*f*
  paraneoplastic cerebellar degeneration
    and, 76–77
  thymoma, 152
malignant hyperthermia (MH), 163–64
maraviroc, 191
Maternal Outcomes and
    Neurodevelopmental Effects of
    Antiepileptic Drugs study, 35–36
mavrilimumab, 244
median nerve, 170. *See also* carpal tunnel
    syndrome
Mediterranean diet, 294–95
medroxyprogesterone acetate, 5
melatonin, 254*t*
memantine, 254*t*
Memory and Cognition in Decreased
    Hypertension substudy, 293

memory concerns in middle age, 291*b*, 292–97
meningiomas, 223
meningitis
  as complication of neuraxial anesthesia, 318
  early neurosyphilis and, 197
  Lyme disease and, 206–7, 211
meningovascular syphilis, 197–98
menopausal hormone therapy (MHT), 288–89
menstrual cycle
  exacerbation of seizures in relation to, 3*b*, 4–5
  menstrually related migraine, 89*b*, 90–92
  tension-type headaches and, 106
mentally challenging activities, brain health and, 297
meralgia paresthetica (lateral femoral cutaneous neuropathy), 179–80
metabolic myopathies, 160, 166
methadone, 270
Methergine, 312–13
methotrexate, 152–53, 153*t*, 244
methoxyflurane halothane, 163–64
methylprednisolone
  for giant cell arteritis, 244
  for MS relapse during pregnancy, 47*b*, 48–49
  in NMOSD management, 62
  for optic neuritis, 231–32
metoprolol, 161
midazolam, 39*b*, 40–41
middle age, memory concerns in, 291*b*, 292–97
midodrine, 254*t*
migraine
  with aura, 81*b*, 82, 83*b*, 84, 87, 95*b*, 96–99, 146
  Chiari malformations and, 125*b*, 127
  complicated, 95*b*, 96*b*, 96–99
  hormonal contraception and, 81*b*, 82–86, 85*t*, 87

menstrually related, 89*b*, 90–92
preeclampsia and, 304
pregnancy and, 86–87
prophylactic medications, 85, 85*t*, 86, 91, 92
reversible cerebral vasoconstriction syndrome and, 312–13
stroke risk and, 82, 87, 97, 146
migrainous infarction (MI), 95*b*, 96*b*, 96–97, 98–99
mild cognitive impairment (MCI), 293
mild neurocognitive disorder (MND), 187–88
mind–body therapies for migraine, 87
MIND diet (Mediterranean–DASH Intervention for Neurodegenerative Delay), 294–95
mini-core disease, 163–64, 166
mirabegron, 254*t*
mirtazapine, 263*t*
miscarriage, 61–62
monoamine oxidase-B inhibitors, 251, 252*t*
monomethyl fumarate (Bafiertam), 50*t*, 52, 52*t*
Montreal Cognitive Assessment, 185*b*, 259*b*
motor symptoms
  of Huntington disease, 259*b*, 260, 263, 263*t*
  of Parkinson's disease, 250–51, 252*t*
multi-core disease, 163–64, 166
multiple sclerosis (MS)
  assisted reproductive technology in, 56
  breastfeeding and, 49, 52*t*, 56, 57
  counseling women on risk in children, 57
  disease-modifying therapy for, 47*b*, 49–55, 50*t*, 52*t*, 57
  hormones and, 208
  NMOSD versus, 60–61
  optic neuritis and, 230*f*, 230–31, 232
  postpartum relapses, 48, 49, 56
  in pregnancy, 47*b*, 48–55, 50*t*, 52*t*, 57
  PRIMS study, 48, 56
  treating relapse during pregnancy, 48–49

muscle relaxants, 164
muscle-specific kinase (MuSK) antibodies, 152, 156
muscular dystrophies (MDs), 159*b*, *See also* genetic myopathies
  congenital, 166
  impact on pregnancy and delivery, 161, 162–64
  management, 161
  overview, 160
myasthenia gravis (MG)
  commonly used medications in, 152–53, 153*t*
  medications exacerbating symptoms, 155*b*, 155
  newborns and, 156, 157
  pregnancy and, 151*b*, 152–56, 153*t*, 157
mycophenolate mofetil
  for MOGAD, 67, 68
  for myasthenia gravis, 152–53, 153*t*
  in NMOSD management, 62–63
myelin oligodendrocyte glycoprotein antibody-associated disease (MOGAD), 65*b*
  clinical features and epidemiology, 66–67
  optic neuritis and, 230–32
  pregnancy and, 67–68
  treatment, 67
myelitis
  in NMOSD, 60–61
  transverse, 60, 66
myelomeningocele, 126
myoclonic jerks, 13–14
myopathies. *See* genetic myopathies
myotonic dystrophy type 1 (DM1), 160, 161, 162, 163–66
myotonic dystrophy type 2 (DM2), 164–65

naproxen, 81*b*, 91
naratriptan, 91, 95*b*
natalizumab (Tysabri), 48, 49, 50*t*, 52*t*, 54–55

needle tip designs for neuraxial anesthesia, 323*f*
nemaline myopathy, 162, 166
neonatal myasthenia gravis, 156, 157
neonatal outcomes
  of cancer treatment, 223–24
  COVID-19 infection during pregnancy and, 214, 215–17
  of genetic myopathies, 165–66
neostigmine, 156
nerve conduction studies (NCS), 176–78, 214–15
neural tube defects (NTDs), 19
neuraxial anesthesia
  Chiari malformations and, 126–27
  complications of, 316–20
  epidural hematoma and, 180–81
  genetic myopathies and, 164
  idiopathic intracranial hypertension and, 116
  needle tip designs for, 323*f*
  postpartum leg weakness and, 179, 180–81, 182
  total spinal block and, 315*b*, 316
neuroacanthocytosis, 280, 281*t*
neuroborreliosis, Lyme, 207, 208–9
neurocognitive impairment disorders among PWH. *See* HIV-associated neurocognitive disorders
neuroleptics, 262, 263*t*, 267–69, 282
neuromodulation devices, 87
neuromodulators, 91
neuromuscular blockade, 164
neuromyelitis optica (NMO), 230–32
neuromyelitis optica spectrum disorders (NMOSD), 59*b*
  AQP4 antibodies and, 60
  clinical clues in, 60–61
  management in pregnancy and postpartum, 62–63
  miscarriage and preeclampsia risks, 61–62
  versus MOGAD, 66
  postpartum relapse, 62

neuropathies. *See also* carpal tunnel
  syndrome
  femoral, 175*b*, 176–78, 181–82
  of lower extremity associated with
    pregnancy and delivery, 179–80
neurosyphilis, 195*b*
  clinical presentation, 197–98
  diagnosis, 199–200
  follow-up after treatment of, 201–2
  overview, 196, 202–3
newborns, myasthenia gravis and, 156, 157
nifedipine, 304
NMDA antagonists, 254*t*, 263*t*
non-arteritic ischemic optic neuropathy
    (NAION), 236–39
non-depolarizing muscle relaxants, 164
non-epileptic seizures (NES), 24
nonmalignant meningioma, 223
nonreactive nontreponemal testing,
    199–200
nonsteroidal anti-inflammatory drugs
    (NSAIDs)
  for migraine, 91, 92, 98
  for reversible cerebral vasoconstriction
    syndrome, 313
nontreponemal testing for syphilis, 199–
    200, 201, 202
norepinephrine, 316
nortriptyline, 108

obesity, brain health and, 293, 294
obstetrical nerve injuries, 176, 179*b*, 179,
    180–81. *See also* femoral neuropathy;
    postpartum leg weakness
obstructive sleep apnea (OSA), 295
obturator neuropathy, 180
occipital nerve blocks, 115
occipital nerve stimulation, 106
occupational therapy, 162, 251
ocrelizumab (Ocrevus), 47*b*, 50*t*, 52*t*, 55
ocular coherence tomography (OCT), 231
ocular manifestations of Lyme disease, 207
ocular syphilis, 197, 198–99, 202

ofatumumab (Kesimpta), 50*t*, 52*t*, 55
olanzapine, 262, 263*t*
onabotulinum toxin A, 86–87, 108
opiates, 98
opicapone, 252*t*
opioids, 164, 270, 313
optical coherence tomography (OCT), 114,
    115
optic nerve fenestration, 115
optic nerve sheath decompression surgery,
    238
optic neuritis (ON), 229*b*, 230*f*
  diagnosis, 230–31
  MOGAD, 66
  in NMOSD, 59*b*, 60
  overview, 230, 236
  treatment, 231–32, 236
oral contraceptive pills (OCPs). *See* family
    planning; hormonal contraception
organ dysfunction in preeclampsia, 302,
    304
orthostatic hypotension, 254, 254*t*
osmotic laxatives, 254*t*
osteoporosis
  overview, 8
  prevention, 9
  risk factors for, 8
  screening for, 9
otosyphilis, 197, 198–99, 202
oxcarbazepine
  bone health and, 8
  for generalized-onset epilepsies, 19
  for migraine, 85*t*
  pregnancy and, 34, 36
  seizures and, 16, 17–18
  status epilepticus during pregnancy and,
    40–41
  for trigeminal neuralgia, 108
oxycodone, 270
oxygen inhalation, 105, 162
oxytocin, migraine and, 91
oxytocin agonists, 91
ozanimod (Zeposia), 50*t*, 52*t*, 53–54

papilledema, 116, 117
paraneoplastic cerebellar degeneration (PCD), 75*b*, 76–77
parathyroid hormone, 8
parkinsonian tremor, 274, 275, 277
Parkinson's disease (PD), 249*b*
  comprehensive management and patient-centered care, 256
  diagnosis, 250, 251
  general discussion, 256–57
  main motor symptoms of, 250
  management of motor symptoms, 251, 252*t*
  non-motor aspects, 250, 254, 254*t*
  overview, 250
  pregnancy and, 251
  pre-motor symptoms, 250
paroxetine, 254*t*
paroxysmal hemicrania, 103*t*
penicillin, 195*b*, 196, 201, 280
pentobarbital, 40–41
people with HIV (PWH). *See* HIV-associated neurocognitive disorders
perimenstrual exacerbation (C1) pattern, catamenial epilepsy, 4, 5
perimenstrual migraine, 89*b*, 90–92
perindopril, 159*b*
periodic limb movements (PLM), 266, 267*t*, 270
periovulatory exacerbation (C2) pattern, catamenial epilepsy, 4, 5
peripartum cardiomyopathy, 161
peripheral nerve blocks without steroids, 108
peripheral nervous system (PNS), 207
peroneal (fibular) neuropathy, 180
Phalen sign, 171
phenobarbital, 8, 34–35, 40–41
phenylephrine, 312–13, 316
phenytoin
  bone health and, 8
  myasthenia gravis and, 155
  oral contraceptive pills and, 34–35

pregnancy and, 40
seizures and, 16, 17–18
for trigeminal neuralgia, 108
pheochromocytoma, 312–13
phosphodiesterase-5 inhibitors, 238
physical activity, brain health and, 295–96
physical therapy, 26, 162, 251
physiologic tremor, 275*b*, 275, 277
pimavanserin, 254*t*
pituitary adenomas, 120, 121
pituitary apoplexy, 119*b*, 120*f*
  anatomy, 121
  clinical features, 121
  definition, 120
  endocrine dysfunction and, 121–22
  overview, 122
  Sheehan syndrome, 120
  treatment, 122
plasma exchange
  for MOGAD, 67
  for myasthenia gravis, 152–53, 153*t*, 157
plasmapheresis
  for anti-NMDA receptor encephalitis, 73–74
  in NMOSD management, 59*b*, 62
  for optic neuritis, 231–32, 236
platelet count, giant cell arteritis and, 242
Plegridy, 49–52
polycystic ovarian syndrome (PCOS), 29*b*–33*b*, 30, 31
polyethylene glycol, 254*t*
polymyalgia rheumatica, 241*b*, 242
polysomnogram, 266
ponesimod (Ponvory), 50*t*, 52*t*, 53–54
positive pressure ventilation, 162
post dural puncture headache (PDPH), 319–20, 321*b*, 322–23, 324
posterior ischemic optic neuropathy (PION), 236–37
posterior pituitary, 121
posterior reversible encephalopathy syndrome (PRES), 307*b*, 308*f*
  clinical features, 308, 309

COVID-19 infection and, 214, 217
pathophysiology, 308–9
versus reversible cerebral vasoconstriction
  syndrome, 312, 313
status epilepticus and, 41
treatment, 309
postmenopausal women, osteoporosis in,
  8, 9
postpartum cerebral venous thrombosis,
  133*b*, 134
postpartum hemorrhage, 165
postpartum leg weakness
  differential diagnosis of, 176–78, 178*b*
  femoral neuropathy, 175*b*, 176–78
  other causes, 180–81, 181*b*
  other lower extremity neuropathies,
    179–80
  overview, 181–82
  risk factors for obstetrical nerve injury,
    179*b*, 179
postpartum relapse
  of MOGAD, 67–68
  of multiple sclerosis, 48, 49, 56
  of neuromyelitis optica spectrum
    disorders, 62
postpartum stroke, 140
post-treatment Lyme disease syndrome
  (PTLDS or chronic Lyme), 205*b*,
  209–11
postural tremor, 274. *See also* essential
  tremor
pramipexole, 252*t*, 265*b*, 269, 270, 271
preconception planning. *See* family
  planning
PREDIMED trial, 294–95
prednisone, 152–53, 153*t*, 244
preeclampsia (PEC), 59*b*, 301*b*, *See also*
  eclampsia
  clinical features, 302, 305
  COVID-19 infection and, 213*b*, 217
  diagnostic criteria, 302, 302*t*, 304
  genetic myopathies and, 163
  migraine and, 86–87

myasthenia gravis and, 155, 157
neuromyelitis optica spectrum disorders
  and, 61–62
pathophysiology, 304
posterior reversible encephalopathy
  syndrome and, 308–9
reversible cerebral vasoconstriction
  syndrome and, 313
treatment, 304, 305
pregabalin, 108, 270, 271
pregnancy. *See also* eclampsia; preeclampsia
  anti-NMDA receptor encephalitis and,
    73–74
  antiseizure medications and, 12–13, 15,
    16, 17*t*, 18–20, 34–31, 40
  arteriovenous malformation and, 129*b*,
    130*f*, 130–32
  brain tumor in, 221*b*, 222–24, 223*f*
  carpal tunnel syndrome and, 169*b*, 170,
    172–73
  cerebral venous thrombosis and, 133*b*,
    134–36
  Chiari malformations, 125*b*, 126–27
  chorea gravidarum in, 279*b*, 280–83,
    281*t*
  clotting factor changes during, 134*f*
  cluster headaches and, 102–6
  COVID-19 infection during, 213*b*,
    214–17
  essential tremor treatment and, 276–77
  genetic myopathies and, 159*b*, 161–67
  Huntington disease and, 261, 262
  hypertension in, 302
  hypertensive disorders of, 215–16, 217,
    302, 302*t*, 304–5
  idiopathic intracranial hypertension in,
    111*b*, 112*f*, 112–17, 113*b*
  ischemic stroke and, 139*b*, 140–42,
    141*f*, 142*f*
  lower extremity neuropathies associated
    with, 179–80
  low-pressure headache in, 321*b*, 322–24,
    323*f*

pregnancy (*cont.*)
  migraine and, 85, 85*t*, 86–87
  MOGAD and, 67–68
  multiple sclerosis in, 47*b*, 48–55, 50*t*, 52*t*, 57
  myasthenia gravis and, 151*b*, 152–56, 153*t*, 157
  neuraxial anesthesia complications, 315*b*, 316–20
  neuromyelitis optica spectrum disorders and, 61–63
  optic neuritis treatment during, 231–32
  Parkinson's disease and, 251
  pituitary apoplexy in, 119*b*, 121, 122
  posterior reversible encephalopathy syndrome in, 307*b*, 308*f*, 308–9
  postpartum leg weakness, 175*b*, 176–82
  restless leg syndrome and, 266, 270, 271
  status epilepticus during, 39*b*, 40–42
  stroke risk and, 146
  syphilis and, 196, 200–1
  tension-type headaches and, 106
  trigeminal neuralgia treatment and, 108
"Pregnancy and Lactation Labeling Rule" (FDA), 34
Pregnancy in Multiple Sclerosis (PRIMS) study, 48, 56
prematurity, genetic myopathies and, 164, 165
presynaptic a₂ antagonist, 263*t*
primary headache disorders, 101*b*
  cluster headaches, 101*b*, 102–6, 103*t*, 108
  overview, 102
  tension-type headache, 102, 103*t*, 106, 107*b*, 108
  trigeminal autonomic cephalgias, 102–6, 103*t*, 105*b*
  trigeminal neuralgia, 103*t*, 105*b*, 107–8
primary syphilis, 196–97, 200
primidone
  bone health and, 8
  for essential tremor, 275–77, 276*t*

progesterone
  brain tumors during pregnancy and, 223
  cyclic lozenges, 5
  seizures and, 4, 30
  stroke risk and, 82
progesterone-only contraception, 86, 97–98
progestin, 288–89
prolactin, 30, 121–22
propofol, 40–41, 116
propranolol
  for essential tremor, 275–77, 276*t*
  for genetic myopathies, 161
  for headache of IIH, 115
  for migraine, 81*b*, 85*t*
  myasthenia gravis and, 155*b*
proteinuria, 302, 304
proton pump inhibitors, 244
proximal weakness, genetic myopathies and, 162–63
pseudodementia, 296
pseudoephedrine, 312–13
pseudoseizures. *See* functional neurologic disorder
psychiatric symptoms of Huntington disease, 260, 263, 263*t*
psychological interventions for functional neurologic disorder, 26
psychosis
  in Huntington disease, 260, 262, 263*t*
  in Parkinson's disease, 254, 254*t*
pulmonary compromise, genetic myopathies and, 159*b*, 162
pulse prophylaxis for migraine, 91
pure menstrual migraine, 90, 91
pyridostigmine, 152–53, 153*t*, 156, 157

quetiapine, 254*t*, 262, 263*t*

radiculoneuritis (Bannwarth syndrome), 206, 207, 211
radiotherapy, 222, 223–24
rapid-acting antihypertensives, 304

346   INDEX

rapid eye movement (REM) sleep behavior disorder, 250, 254*t*

rapid plasma reagin (RPR) test, 195*b*, 202, 203

rasagiline, 252*t*

Rayhill, M., 87

reactive treponemal testing, 199–200

Rebif, 49–52

recombinant follicle-stimulating hormone, 56. *See also* assisted reproductive technology

refractory restless leg syndrome, 265*b*, 269, 270

regional anesthesia. *See* neuraxial anesthesia

remote electrical neuromodulation (REN), 91

renal impairment from preeclampsia, 304

respiratory insufficiency, genetic myopathies and, 159*b*, 162

restless leg syndrome (RLS), 265*b*
  augmentation, 269
  comorbid conditions, 266–67, 268*b*
  diagnosis, 266, 267*t*
  overview, 266, 270–71
  pregnancy and, 266, 270, 271
  primary versus secondary, 266–69
  treatment, 269–70

retroperitoneal hematoma, 178, 182

revascularization procedures, 244

reversible cerebral vasoconstriction syndrome (RCVS), 311*b*
  clinical features, 312, 313
  pathophysiology, 312–13
  status epilepticus and, 41
  treatment, 313

rheumatic fever, 280–82, 281*t*

risperidone, 262, 263*t*

rituximab (Rituxan)
  for anti-NMDA receptor encephalitis, 73–74
  breastfeeding and, 52*t*
  for MOGAD, 67, 68
  in NMOSD management, 62–63
  pregnancy and, 50*t*, 55

rivastigmine, 254*t*

ropinirole, 252*t*, 269, 271

ropivacaine, 319

rotigotine, 252*t*, 269, 271

ruptured arteriovenous malformation, 129*b*, 130*f*, 130, 131–32

safinamide, 252*t*

SARS-CoV-2 infection in pregnancy. *See* COVID-19 infection during pregnancy

satralizumab, 62–63

scoliosis, 166

secondary restless leg syndrome, 266–69

secondary syphilis, 196–97, 200

sedatives, 164

seizures. *See also* antiseizure medications; eclampsia; epilepsy
  absence, 13–14, 15, 16, 17
  assisted reproductive technology and, 35
  in catamenial epilepsy, 3*b*, 4–5
  cerebral venous thrombosis and, 133*b*, 134–35, 136
  in functional neurologic disorder, 24, 25*t*
  in generalized-onset epilepsies, 11*b*, 12, 13–14, 15, 16–17
  generalized tonic–clonic, 13–14, 16, 29*b*, 39*b*, 129*b*, 133*b*
  hormones as influencing, 4, 30
  intravascular injection of local anesthetic and, 319
  in juvenile-onset Huntington disease, 260
  in meningitis, 318
  myasthenia gravis and, 155
  myoclonic jerks, 13–14
  in preeclampsia, 304
  pregnancy and, 19, 34, 39*b*, 40–42
  in PRES, 307*b*, 308, 309
  reversible cerebral vasoconstriction syndrome and, 312, 313

selective serotonin reuptake inhibitors, 254*t*, 263*t*

selegiline, 252t

senna glycoside, 254t

serial CSF evaluations for syphilis, 202

serial lumbar punctures, 115, 117

serofast state, syphilis, 202

serotonergic medications, 312–13

serotonin 1F receptor agonists, 98

serotonin and norepinephrine reuptake inhibitors, 254t, 263t, 312–13

sertraline, 254t, 263t

serum ferritin, 267–69, 271

serum RPR titer for syphilis, 202, 203

sevoflurane, 163–64

sexual dysfunction in Parkinson's disease, 254, 254t

sexually transmitted infections (STIs), 199–200, 201, 203. *See also* syphilis

Sheehan syndrome, 120

short-lasting unilateral neuralgiform headache attacks, 103t

sialorrhea, 254t

sildenafil, 254t

siponimod (Mayzent), 50t, 52t, 53–54

sleep disturbances
  brain health and, 295
  in Parkinson's disease, 250, 254, 254t
  in restless leg syndrome, 266

smoking
  brain health and, 293
  osteoporosis and, 8, 9
  stroke risk and, 82, 83–84, 86, 97–98, 99

social engagement, brain health and, 297

sodium channel agents, 16, 17–18

sotalol, 161

sphenopalatine ganglion stimulation, 106

sphingosine-1-phosphate (S1P) receptor modulators, 49

spinal anesthesia. *See* neuraxial anesthesia

spinal cord infarction, 181

spinal cord injury, 318, 320

spine MRI, 181, 230–31

spontaneous abortion, genetic myopathies and, 165

spot prophylaxis for migraine, 91

status epilepticus (SE)
  absence, 16
  cesarean sections for patients in, 19
  during pregnancy, 39b, 40–42

steroids
  for anti-NMDA receptor encephalitis, 73–74
  for carpal tunnel syndrome, 172–73
  for cluster headaches, 106
  for COVID-19 infection during pregnancy, 213b
  for giant cell arteritis, 244–45
  for low-pressure headache, 324
  for Lyme disease facial palsy versus Bell palsy, 207, 211
  for MOGAD, 67
  for MS relapse during pregnancy, 48–49
  myasthenia gravis and, 152–53, 153t, 156, 157
  in NMOSD management, 62–63
  for obstetrical nerve injury, 179–80
  for optic neuritis, 231–32, 236
  for paraneoplastic cerebellar degeneration, 76–77
  for pituitary apoplexy, 122
  for postpartum MS relapse, 49

steroid-sparing agents, 244–45

stimulant laxatives, 254t

streptococcal infections, 280–82

stress hormones, 296

stroke, 145b, *See also* ischemic stroke
  cerebral venous thrombosis and, 134
  COVID-19 infection during pregnancy and, 214, 216
  hormonal contraception and, 82, 83–84, 97–98
  incidence, 146
  meningovascular syphilis and, 197–98
  migraine treatment and, 98
  migraine with aura and, 82, 84, 97–99
  migrainous infarction, 95b, 96b, 96–97
  overview, 147

in preeclampsia, 304
reversible cerebral vasoconstriction
    syndrome and, 312
risk factors with differential impact in
    women, 146, 147
risk management in women, 146
sex-specific risk factors, 146, 147
subdural hematoma, 322
succinylcholine, 116, 163–64
sumatriptan, 105, 115
surgical management
    of cancer, 222, 223–24
    of carpal tunnel syndrome, 172–73
    of epidural abscess, 318
    of epidural hematoma, 317
    of essential tremor, 275–76
    of ischemic optic neuropathy, 238
    of pituitary apoplexy, 122
    of retroperitoneal hematoma, 178
    of ruptured arteriovenous malformation,
        131f, 131, 132
    of trigeminal neuralgia, 108
swallowing assessments for genetic
    myopathies, 162
Sydenham chorea, 280
sympathomimetics, 238
syphilis, 195b
    changing epidemiology of, 200
    clinical presentation, 196–99
    congenital, 196, 200, 201
    diagnosis, 199–200
    follow-up after treatment of, 201–2
    intrapartum, 196, 200–1
    latent phase, 196–97
    overview, 196, 202–3
    primary, 196–97
    secondary, 196–97
    tertiary, 196–97
    vertical transmission, 201
systemic lupus erythematosus (SLE), 280–
    82, 281t, 312–13
Systolic Blood Pressure Intervention Trial,
    293

tabes dorsalis, 198
tacrolimus, 152–53, 153t, 157, 312–13
tau deposition, 289
telithromycin, 155b
temozolomide, 222
temporal arteritis. *See* giant cell arteritis
temporal artery biopsy, 243f, 243, 244, 245
tenofovir alafenamide, 185b
tension-type headache, 102, 103t, 106,
    107b, 108
teratogenic medication. *See also* topiramate
    for epilepsy, 34–31
    for essential tremor, 276–77
    for idiopathic intracranial hypertension,
        114
    for migraine, 85, 85t, 86–87
    for multiple sclerosis, 53–55
    for myasthenia gravis, 152–53
    for trigeminal neuralgia, 108
teratomas, 72, 73, 74
teriflunomide (Aubagio), 50t, 52t, 54
tertiary syphilis, 196–97
test dose, neuraxial anesthesia, 316, 320
tetrabenazine, 262, 263, 263t, 282
thalamic glioblastoma, 221b, 222–24, 223f
theophylline, 324
thrombectomy, 141
thrombolysis, 141
thunderclap headache, 312, 313
thymoma, 152
Tinel sign, 171
tinnitus, 319, 321b, 322
tirofiba (Aggrastat), 317t
tobacco use. *See* smoking
tocilizumab, 244
topiramate
    bone health and, 8
    for cluster headaches, 106
    for essential tremor, 275–77, 276t
    for generalized-onset epilepsies, 12–13,
        15, 17t, 18
    for idiopathic intracranial hypertension,
        114

topiramate (*cont.*)
  for migraine, 85, 85*t*, 86
  pregnancy and, 34
  status epilepticus during pregnancy
    and, 40–41
total spinal block, 315*b*, 316, 320
transferrin saturation, 267–69, 271
transient neonatal myasthenia gravis, 156,
  157
transmagnetic stimulation, 115
transverse myelitis, 60, 66
tremor
  action, 274–75
  cerebellar, 274, 275, 277
  enhanced physiologic, 275*b*, 275, 277
  essential, 273*b*, 274–77
  in functional neurologic disorder, 24
  head, 275
  kinetic, 274
  parkinsonian, 274, 275, 277
  postural, 274
treponemal testing for syphilis, 199–200,
  201, 202
tricyclic antidepressants, 85*t*, 115
trigeminal autonomic cephalgias (TACs),
  102–6, 103*t*, 105*b*
trigeminal nerve stimulation, 115
trigeminal neuralgia (TN), 103*t*, 105*b*,
  107–8
triptans
  for cluster headaches, 105
  for migraine, 86, 91, 92, 98
  reversible cerebral vasoconstriction
    syndrome and, 312–13

ublituximab (Briumvi), 50*t*, 52*t*, 55
ubrogepant, 91
unruptured arteriovenous malformation,
  130, 132
urinary dysfunction in Parkinson's disease,
  254, 254*t*
U.S. Food and Drug Administration
  (FDA), 34

ustekinumab, 244
uteroplacental ischemia, 304

vaccines
  COVID-19, 216–17
  sex differences in responses to, 208
valbenazine, 262, 263*t*
valproate
  bone health and, 8
  for migraine, 85*t*
  polycystic ovarian syndrome and, 29*b*, 30
  pregnancy and, 34, 35–36
valproic acid
  for cluster headaches, 106
  for generalized-onset epilepsies, 12–13,
    14, 15, 17*t*, 18, 20
  for migraine, 85*t*
  status epilepticus during pregnancy and,
    40–41
Valsalva, 111*b*, 113–14, 125*b*, 126, 127
vascular disorders, in differential diagnosis
  of CG, 280, 281*t*
vascular insufficiency symptoms, 242
vascular risk factors, migraine and, 97–98,
  99
vasoactive agents, 312–13
vasogenic brain edema in PRES, 308–9
vasospasm, 97, 98–99, 312, 313
Venereal Disease Research Laboratory
  (VDRL) test, 195*b*, 199–200
venlafaxine, 85*t*, 254*t*, 263*t*
venous dilatation in low-pressure headache,
  322
venous sinus stenting, 115, 117
verapamil, 85*t*, 106, 313
vertical transmission of syphilis, 201
vesicular monoamine transporter 2
  (VMAT2) inhibitors, 262, 263*t*, 282
video-EEG, 23*b*, 24
vision restoration therapy, 238
visual disturbance
  in posterior reversible encephalopathy
    syndrome, 308

in preeclampsia, 301*b*, 304
in reversible cerebral vasoconstriction
syndrome, 311*b*, 312
visual evoked potentials (VEPs), 231
visual field testing
for idiopathic intracranial hypertension,
114, 115, 117
for optic neuritis, 230–31
vitamin D, 8, 9, 244

warfarin, 283
weight
brain health and, 294–95
in idiopathic intracranial hypertension
treatment, 114
Willis–Ekbom disease. *See* restless leg
syndrome

Wilson disease, 280–82, 281*t*
Woman's Health Initiative study, 8–9
Women's Health Initiative Memory Study
(WHIMS), 288–89
Women's Health Study, 84
Women's Interagency HIV Study, 189
women with epilepsy (WWE). *See* epilepsy
World Health Organization (WHO), 84,
214
wrist, median neuropathy at. *See* carpal
tunnel syndrome

zolmitriptan, 91
zonisamide
bone health and, 8
for generalized-onset epilepsies, 12–13,
15, 17*t*, 18, 19, 20

INDEX 351